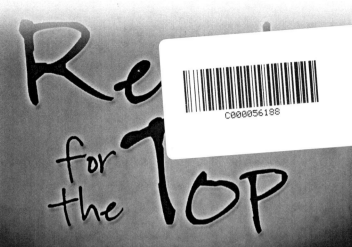

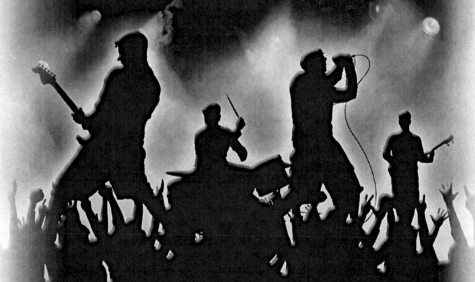

The Musician's Guide to
Health, Wealth, and Success

Timothy Jameson
Doctor of Chiropractic

Vendera
Publishing

ISBN: 978-1-936307-02-9

LC Control No.: 2010920988

Cover & Interior Design: Scribe Freelance | www.scribefreelance.com
Editor: Jaime Vendera

Dr. Jameson is also author of:
The Musicians Health and Wellness Guide
Copyright © 2004 by Timothy Jameson, D.C.

Repetitive Strain Injuries: Alternative Treatments and Prevention
McGraw-Hill; 1 edition (January 11, 1998)
ISBN: 0879838027

DISCLAIMER: The following sections are not intended to treat, diagnose, or prevent any physical, mental or spiritual conditions. Before performing any of the following exercises, or adding any supplements to your diet, please consult your physician.

This book is dedicated to musicians throughout the world who seek to enhance their health, their art, and their life through constant personal improvement.

Many thanks to my editor and encourager, Jaime Vendera, who recognized the need for musicians and vocalists to enhance their health through natural, conservative means.
Jaime, you are a true blessing from God!

Contents

Introduction

ARE YOU CONSIDERING A CAREER AS a musical artist? Are you a musician or vocalist and you feel as if you've reached a plateau in your career? Do you have a nagging injury that is holding you back from excelling in your musicianship? Are you looking for the secret clues that highly successful musicians already know? If you answered YES to any of these questions, then this is the book for you!

This book is a summary of what I have learned about the amazing attributes of the human mind, body, and soul over my 20+year career as a Doctor of Chiropractic and as a musician working week after week as a music director and worship pastor of my church. I have spent many years working intimately with musicians, caring for human beings dealing with injuries, emotional stress, performance stress, and addictions. Through that time, I have thoroughly enjoyed providing wellness enhancement, encouragement, and relief from debilitating injuries. It is one of my greatest joys to see a musician's career saved by chiropractic, and then allowed to flourish due to positive constructive coaching to work on the mental aspect of the game.

I wrote this book in order to present you with the tools that will help you achieve a level of success that you only dreamed for your career. This book will set in motion your desires to reach the top! It is an action-oriented book that will guide you in your path to success. I believe it will be a workbook that you will keep in your travel bag, or next to your bed, so you can constantly revisit your goals, affirmations, and action steps to achieve the results you have desired for your life.

I also created this book so that you can achieve a level of physical wellness that will allow you to perform music, night after night, throughout your entire life. Musicians must care for their bodies to engage in the "sport of music." In the pages that follow you will receive advice in everything from nutritional intake, stretching, physical exercises, breathing techniques, and mental success tips to enhance your musicianship.

I pray that this book encourages you to just "GO FOR IT" and push beyond any fears or self doubts you may have about your musical abilities or physical challenges. So get ready to set a path for greatness, because together, we are going to conquer this trail, although there may be some potholes, diversions, and roadblocks along the way. You can do it! Thank you for reading this book, and may you be blessed by the information presented in the following pages.

DR. TIMOTHY JAMESON

Chapter One

WELLNESS IN THE 21ˢᵀ CENTURY

A wise man should consider that health is the greatest of human blessings, and learn how by his own thought to derive benefit from his illnesses.
HIPPOCRATES (460 BC–377 BC), *Regimen in Health*

Look to your health; and if you have it, praise God and value it next to conscience; for health is the second blessing that we mortals are capable of, a blessing money can't buy.
IZAAK WALTON (1593–1683)

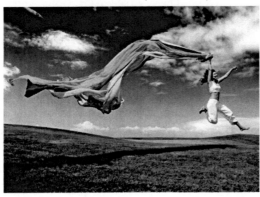

WHAT IS WELLNESS?

The path to your musical success starts with your health. Everyone wants to be healthy, but few people truly understand how to attain health and wellness. If you ask the average person on the street what it means to be healthy, they typically will answer, "when you feel good," or "when I have lots of energy." These nebulous answers get many people in trouble, and years down the line, those exact same people wind up sitting (or lying down) in a doctor's office wondering why they got so sick. This book will give you details on how to enhance your health, creativity, mental prowess, and spiritual nature. These details have been tailored to musicians who have unique needs and concerns, but these are all aspects of health that are critically important not just for the musician, but to every human being.

Whether you're on tour, playing a gig in a local club, or simply learning to play your instrument in your living room, this book will become a companion and helpful resource for you, the musician, who seeks to prevent injuries, enhance your health, and reach your peak performance.

WHY IS WELLNESS IMPORTANT FOR THE MUSICIAN?

As a musician, your music speaks about your current level of wellness. Don't believe me? Listen to the music of musicians who are in deep levels of depression or hold tremendous anger. Their angst pours out of their music and impacts the listener as well. If you've read the *Sing Out Loud* series by Anne Loader McGee and Jaime Vendera, you surely understand how your emotional impact affects the song. The more that I am involved in music as a musician, songwriter, worship leader in a church, and avid listener of the many genres of music, the more I am convinced that music impacts the depths of your heart and soul. Your musical performance therefore is directly related to your current level of your physical, chemical, and emotional health. And that performance impacts countless lives. Imagine that; your performance affects many other listeners' lives…There exists a level of responsibility that most musicians are not really aware of.

Consider the following thought. If you are a songwriter, your writing and composing style is influenced by your own health and wellness, and the health and wellness of those who listen to your music is influenced by your writing and composing style, and the circle continues. So, total health is priority.

If you are a touring musician, you will last only as long as your body and mind are healthy. Lowered levels of health produce interesting effects, including a lowered resistance to colds and flu, sore throats, body aches and strains, back pain, repetitive injuries, impaired digestion, mental sluggishness, and even lost creativity. All this can be avoided with the tools you will learn in the chapters ahead. I will give you practical, real life solutions to what you are facing. You'll want to have this book with you at all times! Stick it in your gig-bag and keep it with you on the road.

Wellness is directly related to mind power and creativity. A healthy body and mind lead to higher levels of musical creativity. How important is the health/creativity connection to the performing artist? Very important! It will determine whether your song gets published or not, whether you can come up with a new lick, whether you'll have lots of fans, as well as determine your endurance while on the road. So you can see that wellness is vitally important to every musician's life.

HOW DOES WELLNESS IMPACT THE ART OF PLAYING AN INSTRUMENT?

We've talked a bit about creativity and mental health, but how about the art of playing music? Your performance is directly proportional to the health of your body. I have often come across

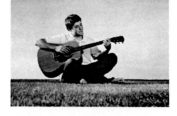

musicians with terrible posture because of years of neglect and ambivalence towards their health. That bad posture is amplified while playing a guitar or while sitting at a piano or whatever instrument they play. They come to me because of the pain they're in, seeking a solution for their health crisis. Because of their level of sickness, their playing ability has been severely hampered, and has affected their live performance.

Many instrumentalists have come to me with problems like tingling and numbness in their hands. Some have to give up playing entirely for a while in order to recover. Do you wonder why your hands are aching and tired after just one hour of playing or why your throat hurts after a few songs? Do you wonder why your neck and shoulders are screaming at you after a two-hour gig? It all comes down to the health and wellness of your "human frame." The good news is that you can take steps to prevent this!

Your overall bodily health will determine your posture, dexterity, and fingering speed. It will also determine your endurance! A healthy body allows for a more erect posture and better integrity of the spinal muscles that create that posture. Higher levels of efficiency of the muscles allow for faster hand movements and more precise fingering on the keyboard or fret board. Body wellness will allow for longer playing sessions as your creativity flows out in abundance.

WHERE DOES HEALTH COME FROM?

That is the question. Here is the challenging answer. *Only YOU can create a healthy body!* It takes incredible fortitude to pursue it. It also takes a decision that the "party life" may just be killing you, and that you need to get back in control of your life again. I am sure there are many teens (and people of all ages) reading this book. READ THIS CAREFULLY, BECAUSE YOUR LIFE DEPENDS UPON IT: Health comes from *within* you, not from pills, potions, and the latest trendy diets and health fads. Health comes from making good, educated decisions that impact every cell of your body. If you keep trying to "get better" by taking pills, you are heading down the path of destruction. So many performing artists had their careers shortened or ended due to addictions to pills that began with a health crisis and led to destruction.

Health and wellness are derived from the following factors: your exercise levels, structural and nervous system health, nutritional health, mental health, spiritual health, the amount of sleep you get, and social factors such as family health, interpersonal relationship health, self-esteem, and connection with a community of like-minded wellness-oriented individuals. Each of these will be discussed in detail as you read further on.

So in other words, health comes only when you decide to "play the game" at full force. Are you ready to step onto the court and take some action? Are you prepared to warm up, work out, and play at 100%? If you answered yes, then the techniques you are about to learn may change your life, your music, and your finances... for the better! But it's not for the timid or the "average person" without drive and dedication, or who wants to live off fast food and sodas. Are you ready to get off the couch and take some action? Are you ready to learn? Let's get started.

BODY, MIND, & SPIRIT

You are composed of three entities that coexist with each other. None of them can function without the other. They are your body, mind, and spirit. Sometimes, they can become out of balance. For example, your spiritual life may seem wonderful, yet you have chronic health problems. You need to find a balance among all three. One of the 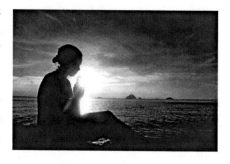 goals of this book is to help bring awareness to areas of your life that are out of balance. Restoring and maintaining balance in these three areas of your life is critically important if you want to achieve the finest musicality possible. Let's discuss each one separately then look at them as a whole.

Your **body** is your physical being. It's your flesh and bones. The health of those flesh and bones are determined by what you feed it. Put in garbage, your flesh and bones will act like garbage. Put in healthy nutritious food, and your flesh and bones will be at their highest level of function. The old saying is absolutely true: Garbage in = Garbage out.

Your **mind** is what controls the functioning of your body. The brain and nervous system are the master controllers of all bodily function. All cells, tissues, organs, muscles, and even blood cells are in direct contact with your nervous system. What you put into your mind determines the health of your body. Again, put in negatively charged data, and your body becomes a haven for sickness and weakness. Put good positive information into your mind and your body becomes equipped to function at peak performance. Your thoughts reflect your outward relationships and help create either negative or positive situations in your life. It is known that how you approach life and how you mentally picture yourself and your life will actually *determine your outcomes in life!* You see yourself as fat – guess what, you'll create it! You see yourself as financially poor – you will create it. See yourself as loving, caring, and compassionate – you will create it. We'll go more into this later on the book.

Your **spirit** is the essence of who you really are as a person. It is my belief that we were all created by a supreme being, and that we each have the potential for spiritual perfection. Now our actions may not be perfect, but the true being within us, our soul, really is perfect. It was designed that way.

I don't believe we are just a combination of chemicals that seeks some type of spiritual existence while living here on earth. What a dismal thought! We are vibrant, creative, spiritual beings that have a predestined purpose for our lives while here on earth. I know there are some of you who are reading this book that in the deepest depths of your understanding, know that you were called to sing and perform throughout the world. You can feel it in every cell of your body and you know it's your life's purpose. Are you preparing your body, mind, and soul for that endeavor, or are you sitting around feeling sorry for yourself because you don't have a record contact and a million fans? Sitting around simply is not an option! You must tap into that perfect spiritual, creative connection that resides in you and allow it to flow like a rushing river.

(Important point – this does not mean YOU are a god, it means you can CONNECT to the all powerful and all knowing God of creation. When you reach that point in life, watch out! You will be unstoppable in your career and in your pursuit of helping others achieve happier lives.)

The exciting part about the body/mind/spirit connection is that once you start working on one area, it impacts the decisions you make about others. For example, if you decide to begin exercising three or four days per week, you begin deciding to eat better because you want to give your body the nutrients required for enhancing your health. Then you start thinking better about yourself, as your mind function enhances because of better oxygenation. Then you begin seeking higher spiritual levels because of all of the above. Can you see how mind/body/spirit interplay with each other? It is similar to three legs of the tripod. All three must function together. When you have all three at optimal levels of wellness, then the world is yours!

THE INSIDE – OUT PHENOMENON

To summarize this wellness concept, it's all about what you put into your mind and body that determines the outcome. In my chiropractic practice, I often tell patients that there exists an "inside-out" phenomenon. Health is created by what you put into your mind and body, and how you feed your soul. This creates the output of what is expressed from your mind/body/soul.

For the musician, this concept is vital to understanding why the wellness movement is so important for you. As you begin enhancing your mind, body, and spirit, your music will follow suit. Your music is a creative expression of the inner you. If you put energy into creating a beautiful YOU, then you will create beautiful music. So let's move onto the next chapter and find out how to do that! So, it's time to put all my words into action and begin learning how to change the mind/body/soul connection for the better.

Chapter Two

WELLNESS FOR THE BODY – PART I – EXERCISE

My heart, which is so full to overflowing, has often been solaced and refreshed by music when sick and weary.
MARTIN LUTHER *(1483 - 1546)*

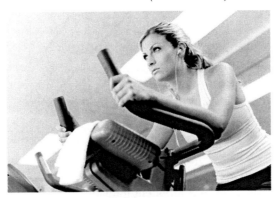

PHYSICAL ACTIVITY – EXERCISE, EXERCISE, EXERCISE!

Have you ever considered yourself an athlete? Well, you are! Hard to believe, isn't it? Remember this statement – ALL MUSICIANS ARE ATHLETES! If you are an instrumentalist, you are an athlete, if you are a singer, you are an athlete – except you don't have to prepare for hurdles, rounding the bases, or shooting a three-pointer. What you *do* need to prepare for is tens of thousands of hand movements, hundreds of repetitive shoulder and elbow motions, constant spinal muscle activity, and continual legwork from moving around the stage or playing the drums. And for singers, who use one of the most amazing instruments of all – the human vocal cords, you are working dynamic intricate systems of muscles within your throat. Every time you play your instrument, the brain is coordinating all this muscle movement to allow your outward expression. Just like an athlete trains and prepares the body in advance of the sporting activity, the musician must do the same to prevent injuries and to enhance endurance.

If you're physically fit and have put in the proper exercise and techniques to enhance and build your muscular systems to respond to the tasks, then these movements are usually no problem and your body will respond well to your brain's commands for movement. Here's the question though. How many musicians are physically fit and at their peak physical performance while playing? I doubt it is more than 20% of the musician population. And I would suspect it is much less than that.

So if you want to achieve total wellness, then guess what? That's right – it's time to get off the couch and begin a total body-training regimen. That doesn't mean you have to begin training at the gym for two hours a day. It does mean that you need to begin thinking differently and integrating an exercise program into your life that occurs at least four to five days per week.

An exercise program for a musician should be made up of four major components:

1) A regular stretching routine, particularly before playing your instrument.
2) An aerobic exercise routine.
3) A large muscle group exercise training program for chest, back, and legs.
4) A small muscle group exercise program, specifically tailored for the instrument you are playing.

Let us take a look at each component individually:

STRETCHING

Maintaining and enhancing flexibility is incredibly important for a musician. Attempting to play an instrument with stiff, tight, cold muscles and joints can make you more susceptible to injury and will definitely slow you down in your speed and acuity. A basic stretching regimen before you play can be a simple task to enhance your stage performance, prevent injury, and improve your flexibility and endurance. Stretching offers the following benefits:

1) Increases your range of motion
2) Maintains joint mobility
3) Relaxes tightened muscles
4) Can increase circulation
5) Prepares the structural system for work
6) Mentally prepares you for the task at hand
7) Enhances the mind-body connection

The purpose of the exercises recommended here are to introduce a very simple stretching program that covers many of the major muscle groups used by most instrumentalists/vocalists. Should you want to investigate stretching more, particularly for very specific muscle groups, consider reading the books recommended at the end of this section. For vocalists, I highly recommend the book *Raise Your Voice Second Edition* by Jaime Vendera, which offers specific stretches and routines to release tension in the throat.

Some general rules about stretching:

1) Stretching should be a very gentle, slow moving activity. Do not bounce back and forth or forcibly thrust your body into these positions. You can injure yourself if you do these wrong.

2) Hold each stretch for about 15 to 20 seconds (or longer if you're capable) and exhale as your body elongates into that position.

3) Use your breathing to enhance the stretch. Inhale before your stretch, and then exhale as you go into the stretch. If you are going to repeat the stretch, release the tension, inhale again, and then exhale as you attempt to go deeper into the stretch.

4) Stretching should feel good, yet you will feel your body's tension areas. Stretching should not be painful – if you feel pain, let off the stretch and take it slower. Repeated pain patterns can indicate joint swelling, muscle spasm, or other musculoskeletal malady. Consider seeking a health care practitioner should the pain continue.

(Thanks to my daughter Jillian for modeling these exercises!)

THE HEAD/NECK REGION

In these stretching examples, the muscles of the neck are gently stretched. You can aid in the movement of your neck by GENTLY adding a little pressure towards the end range of motion with your hands. IF YOU FEEL DIZZY DOING THESE STRETCHES, STOP IMMEDIATELY! It could indicate arterial problems in your 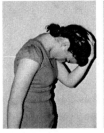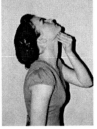 neck or spinal misalignments in your cervical spine that need attention right way.

The first two stretches are for the neck flexors (forward motion) and neck extensors (backward motion). Gently tug forward on the top of the head as you go forward. As you stretch backward into extension, gently push upward on the lower aspect of the jaw (be careful if you have jaw issues) to increase your extension. For vocalists, the gentle neck extension stretch is really important to release tension in the anterior neck muscles.

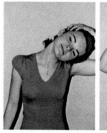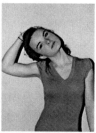

The photos to the left, show left and right lateral neck bending stretches. Gently tug your head toward the side and allow the opposite side neck muscles to stretch.

The neck rotation stretches shown in the photos below help to maintain your neck mobility and stretch both the anterior and posterior neck muscles. Very gently tug on the jaw line as you pull your head so you are looking over your shoulder.

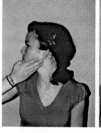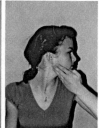

Obviously, everyone is going to have differing abilities at these stretches. The more difficulty you have with them, the more spinal stress, muscular imbalance and tension, and possibly arthritis you are suffering from. Work with your neck over a period of weeks to enhance mobility, and if you are having continued difficulties, seek the aid of a chiropractor to diagnose underlying spine disorders.

THE SHOULDER AND UPPER ARM REGION

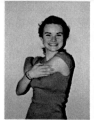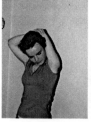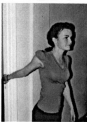

The shoulder and arm region need to be stretched above, forward, and back to involve all the major muscle groups. I find that most instrumentalists have very tense chest muscles, so I would highly recommend you spend some time on the shoulder and chest stretches shown above. The stretch in the above picture on the left works the posterior shoulder muscles, shoulder blade muscles and the muscles between the shoulder blade and spine. The center photo shows a stretch, which works the latissimus muscle, the shoulder blade muscles, and the rib cage muscles. The stretch in the above photo on the right works the chest muscles. Alternate this stretch by grabbing onto the edge of a doorway as shown, first keeping your arm parallel to the floor, then moving the arm slowly up the door frame in small intervals until it is over your head. Hold each interval stretch for 20 to 30 seconds. This will involve all the fibers of the pectoralis muscles that control arm forward motion.

THE FOREARM/HAND REGION

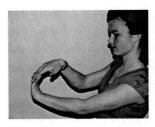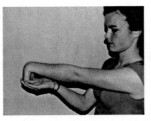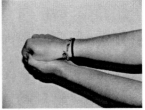

Needless to say, if you're playing instruments, your hands must be prepared for the work ahead. These are some simple stretches to enhance your hand and finger flexibility. The stretch on the above left picture elongates the finger flexor muscles from the hands to the forearms. These are really important to stretch, as you are constantly using them in playing music. The center picture demonstrates a stretch that is simply going the opposite direction and stretching the hand extensors. You'll feel this in your forearm as well. Finally, the above picture on the right is a stretch to help elongate the muscles that work the thumb. Put your thumb inside your hand and gently pull the hand towards the pinky side. You'll feel a stretch go up the thumb-side of the arm. In the photos above, the top hand is the one being stretched. The bottom hand is assisting the motion.

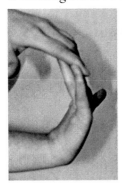

The hands and fingers also benefit from stretching, especially for musicians who perform thousands of hand and finger motions during a concert. All of these stretches should become part of your regular routine in preparation for a gig. Now onto finger stretches.

The first finger stretch shown in the left picture is a simple extension stretch of the entire palm and the finger flexors. Grab on to the ends of the fingers and gently tug backwards. You will feel a stretch in the fingers themselves, then into the palm, and finally the wrist.

Next, let's work the small muscles that move the fingers both medially and laterally by stretching between each finger as shown to the right. Again –

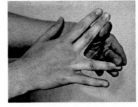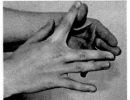

gentleness is the key to these stretches. Stretch each web.

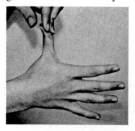
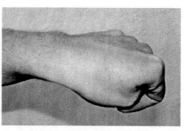

To stretch the thumb region, open the hand up as the picture on the left shows, grabbing the tip of the thumb and pulling it back. You can impact different muscles by slightly rotating the thumb forward and stretching, then pulling the thumb back and stretching it again. The photo on the above right shows the thumb being pulled inward. Grab hold of the thumb with your fingers and contract the wrist muscles away from the thumb side. You should feel a stretch that goes from the thumb up the side of the forearm. (By the way, if any of these finger stretches cause pain, it could indicate joint problems or inflammation in the tendon sheaths or coverings. Discontinue and seek the help of a chiropractor to determine the cause of the pain.)

THE TRUNK / TORSO REGION

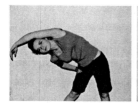
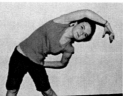

All instrumentalists use their trunk region for stabilization and relaying force from the torso into the arms. Vocalists need incredible torso and diaphragmatic control, so preparing these muscles and creating motion in the joints in advance helps to improve upon your abilities. Elongating and stretching these muscles are really important for everyone from drummers, vocalists, and guitarists, to pianists.

The side stretches above involve lateral torso bending. This opens up the rib cage, releases tensions in the muscles between the ribs, and also benefits by stretching the shoulder muscles. This stretch is great for vocalists, as it releases tensions in the torso, and allows improved rib cage expansion.

The two stretches depicted to the right are for flexion and extension of the spine. The forward flexion stretch, in the first picture to the right, releases tension in the lower back, the back of your upper legs, and glutes. The extension stretch in the second picture to the right helps to release abdominal

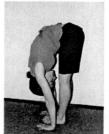
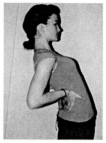

tension, as well as lower chest and diaphragmatic tension. If you have preexisting back problems, please be careful with these stretches. If they cause pain in your spine as you perform them, stop the stretch. And, yes, Jillian in the photos is very flexible, but she is a dancer – you may not be able to achieve the level of flexibility in your stretching that she does – that's ok. Take it at your own pace.

THE LEGS

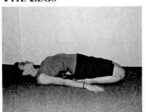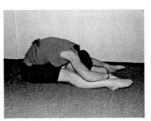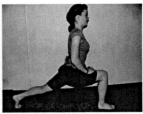

Whether you are a guitarist playing for a couple of hours or a drummer using repetitive foot action upon the bass pedals, you need to prepare your legs like an Olympic hurdles athlete preparers for the race.

Fortunately, Jillian can bend back extremely far to do the quadriceps stretch shown in the above left photo. Most people will not be able to go that far back. Take this slowly and go back as much as you can. Support your upper body with your arms as you bend back. To stretch you ankles as well, tuck them under your buttocks – just be careful. If you have a history of bad ankle sprains, I wouldn't recommend this. Another easier option is to hold onto a chair with one hand, and with the opposite hand and leg, pull the leg back and upward by grasping on to the ankle. This also stretches the quadriceps.

The center photo shows a simple forward flexion stretch for the hamstrings, gluteals, and lower back. First, point the toes straightforward with the legs touching in the middle. Reach towards the toes as far as you can and slowly stretch forward as you exhale. Then separate the legs and continue stretching alternately to one leg, towards the middle, then towards the opposite leg. This helps isolate the hamstring and back muscles.

The stretch on the far right in the photo up above is a lunge-style stretch that helps release tension in a number of muscle groups. It helps stretch the hip flexors (Iliopsoas), the quads, hams, and calves. It's an excellent stretch to release tensions throughout the leg. If you only have a few minutes to warm up, this is the stretch to do. Just perform the stretch on both sides. Allow the torso to sink down toward the floor.

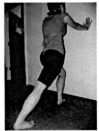

Finally, this last stretch in the picture directly to the right is important to release tensions in the calf. Alternate this stretch by first keeping your knee locked and leg straight. Keep your heel on the floor as you lean forward. Then, bend the knee, keeping the heel on the ground, and lower the knee down until you feel a stretch lower in the calf. This works different muscle groups near the Achilles tendon attachments that are often missed in most stretching programs.

This stretching regimen should be an adequate starting place. For further information about stretching I recommend the following books:

DR. J'S RECOMMENDED BOOKS FOR STRETCHING:

Stretching: 20th Anniversary Revised Edition by Bob Anderson, Jean Anderson; Publisher: Shelter Publications, Incorporated
Pub. Date: January 2000; ISBN-13: 9780936070223

The Genius of Flexibility: The Smart Way to Stretch and Strengthen Your Body by Bob Cooley; Publisher: Simon & Schuster Adult Publishing Group
Pub. Date: August 2005; ISBN-13: 9780743270878

Raise Your Voice 2nd Edition by Jaime Vendera; Publisher: The Voice Connection/Vendera Publishing;
Pub. Date: November 2, 2007; ISBN-10: 0974941158

The Wharton's Stretch Book by Jim Wharton, Phil Wharton; Publisher: Crown Publishing Group
Pub. Date: July 1996; ISBN-13: 9780812926231

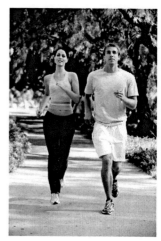

AEROBIC EXERCISE

You might think to yourself, "I'm just sitting here playing my guitar, why is it important for me to get into aerobic shape?" The answer is simple. For you to express yourself and have the highest creativity and brain function, you need optimum oxygenation of your brain. Aerobic exercise and conditioning enhances oxygenation of the tissues, efficiency of the heart muscle, and increases your metabolic rate. Brain

2) Begin enhancing your workout schedule so that you are pushing your heart muscle more intensely per session. Add in more strenuous activities like stair climbing, jumping rope, jumping on a rebounder, and cardio programs you can purchase on DVD that take you through a complete routine that pushes you beyond your current capabilities. Just remember – there is always a step higher in health than you currently have attained!

3) For those who really enjoy weight training, you can also build heart muscle strength by taking less time between sets. I guarantee that if you simply take a minute off between each set of weight training exercises you will see a dramatic change in your heart rate.

4) Just as with the sedentary musician, there's nothing better to help you stay accountable and consistent like a coach – whether it be a friend who will keep you on your routine, or a personal trainer who can take you to the next level in health and fitness.

For the Seasoned Athletic Musician (you currently are in an active program, five days per week, and are in peak aerobic health)

1) Congratulations! You are in the top 5% of your field as far as aerobic health goes. But don't forget – health does not come from exercise alone. I've found that many highly trained athletes are engrossed in their training program, forgetting that health is also dependent upon your nutrition, neurological, social, and mental well-being. Working out five times per week intensively, but yet holding grudges and hatred within your soul will still lead to poor overall health. Begin working on the "whole package."

2) As I said before, there is never a ceiling at cardiac health. Ask an Olympian if he/she can do better, and they will always say "yes." Begin taking notes of your achievement levels, take your pulse at peak aerobic performance, and then mark down your respiratory rate per minute. (The amount of breaths you take each minute.) Begin working at enhancing these areas to increase efficiency of these organs during aerobic exercise. Enhance the awareness of your body, and then work at improving your efficiency.

3) And yes, just like in the other categories – if you don't have a coach, you need one. If you have reached this level of fitness, most likely you have investigated different avenues of workout

regimens. Seek the aid of one or more experts in the field to take you to a new level.

4) Change your routine! Your body will adapt – even to the most difficult aerobic routines. At least two or three times per year, you should change your aerobic workout regimen. If you're running 45 minutes per day, then go to swimming 30 minutes per day and build your endurance in that discipline. Then consider biking. You are a triathlete in training!

PURPOSE

All this exercise gets back to our primary purpose- building our machine to enhance performance and endurance. If you want to perform throughout the world, your endurance will be tested. Those who are at the high level of aerobic training will meet the demands on their bodies with prolonged touring and gigging.

Special Note: Training While On Tour

So, you've prepared your body to go on a world tour! Congratulations. The tour begins…NOW WHAT? Do you just stop and hope the training paid off? That's the worst thing you could do. You don't quit practicing guitar, writing music, or quit your vocal routine when on tour, do you? I hope not. Your body will lose its capabilities quickly as the demand upon it diminishes. You've invested all that time into your body, now you must continue working it while on tour.

Sure, it's tough, whether you're on the tour bus or flying in planes all over the place – but it comes down to priorities and discipline. You will need to sit down and **plan your day** so you can add in continued exercise during your tour. A half-hour workout five days a week will keep you in top shape to handle all the stresses of touring. Movement of your muscles is so important, particularly with long flights or bus rides. Exercise will maintain your flexibility and increase oxygenation of the muscles that have become congested from these cramped environments.

For some musicians planning your day means sitting down with your tour manager and insisting on time for exercise. Don't let him/her run your life. You are in control of your life – create your vision and go for it. That's what brought you on tour in the first place! And hey, if you schedule time for exercise, then that means the rest of your band should have the time too! Get them involved! They can always keep a tour diary and schedule their training time every day on their diary in between interviews, etc.

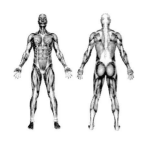

MAJOR MUSCLE GROUP TRAINING

I am hoping you've started to include stretching and cardio into your tour diary. But I need to let you know that there is more work to be done than stretching and aerobic exercise. You must also consider strength training of the major muscle groups. Your major muscle groups, such as the core muscles that stabilize your body, the spinal erectors, the abdominals, the pectoralis (chest) muscles, the quadriceps and hamstrings (thighs), the glutes and the lower leg muscles, all have an impact on your ability to play at full intensity.

Exercising these groups of muscles through intentional weekly programs is another important aspect of building your music machine – your body that intertwines with the instrument through a dynamic interplay.

If you are already performing the aerobic activities mentioned under the previous heading, you are working many of these muscle groups through those workouts. For example, in stair climbing, you're really working the quads and hamstrings in your legs, and lower leg muscles – even the muscles in the feet! They are getting some great repetitive activity training – great for drummers! If you are swimming, you are using every core muscle, from your abs to the glutes to the chest and back muscles to the legs. Swimming is a great exercise for string players such as guitarists, cello players, upright bass players – those who really use their upper body to impart movement into their instrument. And walking works all the major muscle groups!

For those of you who want to enhance the performance of your muscles even more, the next step is beginning a weight training regimen in conjunction with aerobic training. The basic premise of weight training is that you are working a muscle to withstand greater and prolonged loads by increasing and enlarging the number of muscle fibers for greater efficiency. Greater efficiency means that you perform less work to perform a task, such as repetitive kicking the bass drum, or strumming the guitar.

I have found that one of the major reasons for injury in performing artists is simply the fact that the person's muscular system is inadequately trained for the repetitive muscle movements needed for playing music. An untrained muscle will simply not hold up over a period of time of repetitive motor tasks. It will begin to first develop what are called microtears, where the little muscle filaments will begin to tear apart due to the stress imposed upon them by repetitive actions, and then the muscle's attachments to the tendons that connect the muscles to the bones will begin to inflame and tear. This is what causes the pain!

Do you realize how many hundreds of times you strum a guitar in just one song? How about how many movements of your upper body are involved in moving the bow in playing a Mozart piece on the violin or cello? If you are a serious musician, you will discipline yourself to begin training your entire body for the Olympic task of playing an instrument.

A mistake many people make when beginning muscle training is to over-train the muscle. This means that most people do not give the muscle a couple of days to heal after the workout training session. Many people think that if they exercise a muscle group, for example the chest, every day they will get better results. This is far from the truth – muscles need healing after a vigorous strength training session. For this reason, many personal trainers offer a three day program of working chest muscles and triceps the first day, back muscles and biceps the second day, and finally legs and abs on the third day. This process is then repeated again. This way, you're training the same body part a maximum of two times in one week, allowing healing time for the muscles, and maximal results from your training schedule.

If you would like to investigate muscle-training routines in more depth, I would recommend the following books:

DR. J'S RECOMMENDED BOOKS FOR WEIGHT TRAINING:

Weight Training Workouts that Work
by James Orvis; Ideal
Pub. Date: April 1, 2000; ISBN-10: 0967518822

Men's Health Home Workout Bible
by Lou Schuler; Rodale Books
Pub. Date: November 9, 2002; ISBN-10: 1579546579

Strength Training for Women
by Joan Pagano; DK ADULT
Pub. Date: December 27, 2004; ISBN-10: 0756605954

(All recommended books can be quickly found by visiting my website www.musicianshealth.com and clicking on the "recommended books" tab)

THE CORE MUSCLES

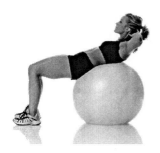

All instrumentalists use major muscle groups to physically control their musical instrument, to artistically express themselves, and to create force to translate onto the instrument's surface, strings, fret board, bass drum pedals or keys. Your power center for all movement is derived from your core muscles, such as your abdominals, pelvic muscles, and back muscles. These muscles must be adequately trained and balanced to play your musical instrument effectively and with the least effort possible.

The buzzwords in physical training regimens lately are "train the core muscles." For the average person, this has no meaning, and leaves most people bewildered at where to begin. The core muscles provide balance, symmetry, and power to your body's structural system surrounding your core – the area between your diaphragm, pelvis and abdomen. The core muscles surround your spine and encase your abdominal organs. Training the core muscles provides the following benefits:

1) Increased efficiency of body movement
2) Improved balance
3) Improved flexibility of the trunk region
4) Improved mind-body connection to your core region
5) Improved diaphragmatic control – impacting breathing – very important for vocalists.
6) Enhanced stabilization of the spine and decreased pressure upon the spinal discs to ensure a healthier structure and nervous system.

The core muscles can be exercised in a number of ways. There are training regimens using medicine balls, balance balls, wobble boards, and other balance products. But even standard exercises such as squats, abdominal workouts, push-ups, and hip flexor exercises can improve the core muscle groups. For those interested in learning more about core strengthening, I would suggest the following excellent books:

DR. J'S RECOMMENDED BOOKS FOR CORE STRENGTHENING:

The Core Strength Workout: Get Flat Abs and a Healthy Back by Karon Karter; Fair Winds Press
Pub. Date: April 4, 2004; ISBN-10: 1592330576

Ultimate Core Ball Workout: Strengthening and Sculpting Exercises with Over 200 Step-by-Step Photos by Jeanine Detz; Ulysses Press Pub. Date: April 10, 2005; ISBN-10: 1569754683

Solid to the Core: Simple Exercises to Increase Core Strength And Flexibility by Janique Farand-taylor; New Harbinger Publications;
1 edition: April 2006; ISBN-10: 1572244305

(All recommended books can be quickly found by visiting my website www.musicianshealth.com and clicking on the "recommended books" tab)

SMALL MUSCLE GROUP TRAINING

For the musician, the small muscles of the forearms and hands are just as important as the large muscles of the torso. I often recommend wrist flexion/extension exercises with three to five pound dumbbells. Try the following exercises:

Forearm flexion exercises working the hand flexors. . . . Start with the hand extended with a lightweight dumbbell. . .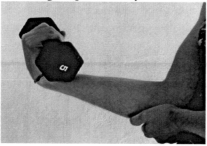

. . . And then pull the weight upwards so your wrist bends towards you.

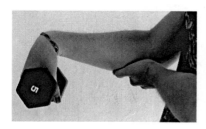

Forearm extension exercises . . .

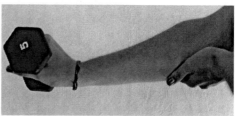

Hold the dumbbell with palm down towards the floor. Bend the wrist upward while supporting your elbow, as in the picture above.

It is also important to strengthen the intrinsic muscles of the hand, which are used for gripping, playing chords, picking strings, holding drumsticks, generally for playing the instrument. I often suggest buying some hand putty. You can find this in most sporting goods stores. The putty of malleable and you simply grip it in the palm of your hand, and then squeeze/release the putty repetitively, to work the different muscles. Another option is a grip strength builder that you can also find in most sporting goods stores.

Don't forget about the finger extensor muscles, which give you the ability to stretch out the hand and fingers. Simply using one or two rubber bands to work the finger extensor muscles can powerfully enhance your dexterity. Start with the rubber bands wrapped around your fingers – near the last joint, and then simply expand your hand open so you have resistance on the rubber band. Repeat at least ten times or until your muscles fatigue.

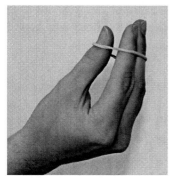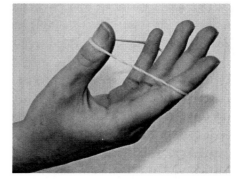

Another great option for finger muscle strengthening are Fingerweights™ by the Fingerweight Corporation. These are great muscle strengtheners that you can actually wear while playing your instrument. You build strength as you play, and when you take them off, you'll find your finger speed will increase as well. These can be purchased through my website, www.musicianshealth.com or directly at www.finger-weights.com.

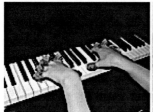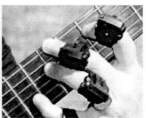

Fingerweights®

Small muscle group training should be performed about every two to three days, depending upon how vigorous you plan to train them. If you are an instrumentalist, then I would not recommend too vigorous a training program, as you could fatigue the muscles enough to impact your playing ability afterwards. If you're working the small muscle groups about three times per week, then you're on a good routine to keep yourself strong and free from injury.

"Wow, do you expect me to be in the gym all day long?"

Not exactly, but I personally understand that after reading these suggestions, it can become intimidating to even begin an exercise program. How could you possibly do all of these exercises and keep up with your regular daily activities and responsibilities? I don't expect you to do each exercise every day. In fact, they should be spread out. Here are some suggestions for you so you can see how it would work. Of course, I would recommend you speak with a personal trainer, your chiropractor or your physician to determine the workout routine that is correct for you. This is simply an example to show you how this complete system would be integrated together on a weekly basis.

Monday: 20 minute aerobics, exercise legs, abs, wrist extensors, exercise ball training

Tuesday: 20-minute aerobics, exercise chest, triceps, wrist flexors

Wednesday: 20-minute aerobics, exercise back, biceps, hand extensors, exercise ball

Thursday, 30 to 40-minute aerobic training, neck shoulder exercises

Friday: Begin system again: 20-minute aerobics, exercise legs, abs, wrist extensors, etc.

Saturday/Sunday – Take these days off. You can alternate the days off with one during the week, and working out Saturday instead. Just commit to five days per week for optimum training levels.

"But I'm a vocalist – how do I exercise?"

Let's consider what is needed in the health of a vocalist: great lung capacity, diaphragm strength (and relaxation), neck, torso, and abdominal strength, endurance, relaxed postural muscles, and with that a healthy upright posture. Now, let's examine each area and how we can improve upon your vocal abilities, simply by implementing a great exercise routine specific to your unique needs.

Your lung capacity is a direct result of your aerobic conditioning, the health of your structure including the spine, the rib cage, the shoulder articulations such as between the collarbone and sternum, your diaphragm control, and your breathing techniques. I already mentioned how to improve aerobic health. Let's get this completely clear: If you are a vocalist – you MUST improve your aerobic health. I would highly recommend exercises that really push your heart and lungs to their maximum level for your age range. You will notice longer note duration, less windedness between long passages, and overall better endurance to last through long concerts.

The structural components I mentioned above, such as the health of your spine, rib cage, articulations with the shoulders should best be evaluated by a Doctor of Chiropractic who is trained to detect misalignments, malfunction, blockages, and tension in those joints and surrounding muscles. On your own, though, you can begin breathing exercises that focus on rib cage expansion and contraction, diaphragm expansion and relaxation, and relaxation of overall upper torso movement with breathing. I highly recommend the following books for vocalists looking to enhance their breathing abilities:

DR. J'S RECOMMENDED BOOKS ON BREATHING:

The Ultimate Breathing Workout
by Jaime Vendera/Vendera Publishing;
Pub. Date: January 1, 2005; ISBN-10: 097494114X

The Tao of Natural Breathing: For Health, Well-Being, and Inner Growth by Dennis Lewis; Rodmell Press;
Revised edition: March 2, 2006; ISBN-10: 193048514X

The Art of Breathing: 6 Simple Lessons to Improve Performance, Health, and Well-Being
by Nancy Zi; Frog Books;
Pub Date: August 28, 2000; ISBN-10: 1583940340

(All recommended books can be quickly found by visiting my website www.musicianshealth.com and clicking on the "recommended books" tab

The health of the neck and shoulder muscles are very important for the vocalist as is the overall posture that you hold your upper body. I will write more on the importance of good posture later in the book, but let's just say that if your posture is bad, your vocal ability is going to be less than optimum. In fact, I would go so far as to say that poor posture combined with spinal stress and nerve stress will not only limit your vocal abilities, but can lead you down a road of vocal irritation, development of polyps, and other vocal cord conditions, which could limit your vocal career. I can't say enough about how important this subject is. Muscular training in both posterior and anterior neck strength, along with shoulder strength, upper back strength, chest strength, and abdominal strength are all vitally important to the vocalist.

If you need a great vocal strength-training program, go to the website, www.venderapublishing.com and check out their vocal product line. In essence, the vocal performer's training routine should be similar to the one mentioned above. I would add the breathing dynamics taught in the books mentioned, along with specific training techniques from Vendera Publishing.

"WHAT IF I'M IN PAIN? SHOULD I CONTINUE TO EXERCISE?"

Pain is a subjective feeling. That means that it has to do with your mental, emotional, chemical, and physical well-being. When beginning an exercise program, most people go through occasional bouts of discomfort, soreness, and pain. It's an inherent part of the process of your body adapting to the forces being placed upon it. Your muscles will produce lactic acid as they are worked hard, producing soreness. Your joints could even get a little sore as you push them beyond their normal routines.

Everyone knows that feeling of soreness after a workout – sometimes for two or three days afterwards. (By the way, that's the reason you don't want to retrain a muscle for two or three days after exercising it – it needs time to heal after a hard workout.) That soreness after your workout is a sign that your body is healing and strengthening.

But, you should also know that experiencing unusual or excruciating pain during your workout is NOT normal. Something may be wrong with your structural or muscular system and a physical check up by a chiropractor should occur at that time. I recommend a Doctor of Chiropractic because the M.D. will just recommend meds and tell you to come back if the pain doesn't subside. Now I'm sure some of you who are reading this book have great family doctors who you trust. That's great! Just realize medicine has its limitations, and dealing with musculoskeletal strain and injuries is definitely not something that medicine does well with. In most cases the M.D. will refer you to a chiropractor or physical therapist for these conditions.

If you try to exercise through the pain, you most likely will harm yourself even more. You can cause injuries such as muscle tears, muscle-tendon junction inflammation, microtears, and tendon-bone junction irritation. Pain is a serious warning sign. Don't ignore the message – and don't take medication to stop the pain and then try to exercise! Without the pain signals, you will have no way of telling if or how much you are injuring yourself.

I believe I've covered enough about exercise in this chapter. To further your knowledge on this subject, I encourage you to purchase one or more of the recommended books that grab your interest. Knowledge is POWER! Let's now move on to improving the body by other means. Our next stop: Nutrition.

Chapter Three

WELLNESS FOR THE BODY – PART II – NUTRITION

YOU CAN AND WILL IMPROVE YOUR music machine by stretching, cardio, and weight training. But there are other considerations to building a fit machine as well, such as sleep, hydration, and nutrition. Bring them all together and you will not only become fit for music, but fit for life as well. Let's begin with nutrition.

NUTRITIONAL WELLNESS

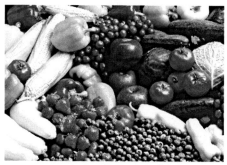

If you are new to nutritional concepts, I recommend that you begin researching in the library or check out the recommended books listed below regarding the basic knowledge of nutrition. For example, you will need to know the difference between carbohydrates, proteins, and fats. I will not spend the time on those basic differences here, but will emphasize the importance of a good diet, supplementation, and water intake. I will also mention the importance of weight loss for the overweight and obese musician. Before moving on, here are few books that I highly recommend reading:

DR. J'S RECOMMENDED BOOKS ON NUTRITION:

Nancy Clark's Sports Nutrition Guidebook
by Nancy Clark: Human Kinetics Publishers;
4th edition: March 14, 2008; ISBN-10: 0736074155

Nutrition Almanac by John Kirschmann; McGraw-Hill;
6th edition: December 21, 2006; ISBN-10: 0071436588

*(All recommended books can be quickly found by visiting my website
www.musicianshealth.com and clicking on the "recommended books" tab*

THE MUSICIAN'S DIET

What is a musician to eat? Let's start with what NOT to eat. Here are some foods that will destroy your health: French fries, chips, sodas, and most fast food. And don't forget the "three evil whites:" white sugar, white flour, and white salt. (The three evil whites is the subject of an entirely different book, which I urge you to research on your own. Once you begin researching all three, you'll quickly learn about their energy leaching properties.)

You must begin treating your body like a temple and not the local garbage dump. It's all about making good decisions. Do you want to have energy to spare when playing that difficult piece of music? Or do you want to feel sluggish, tired, and fatigued when being expected to play 64th notes? Your nutritional intake affects your musicality. Put good nutritious foods into your body that will energize your cells and the effects will be spectacular on your performance and endurance. Keep on reading and you'll learn what these good nutrients are.

It is easy for the tour bus driver to pull off the road at a drive-through fast food restaurant. It is just as easy for that driver to pull off at a restaurant where the musicians can pick up a salad with their meal and eat more nutritious foods. Make your food choices known to your crew and fellow band members so you don't wind up eating junk every day that will destroy your performance ability. You are in control of your body – don't allow others to bring your health and wellness quotient down because of poor choices.

WHERE TO START

All of our bodies are made differently. There is not one diet that will be perfect for everyone, thus I cannot give generalized statements on what types of foods to eat. I am a firm believer that we are all made differently, from different metabolic types, to different blood types. There is not one eating plan that will work across the board for every human being because we are all inherently physiologically different. There are some people who need more protein than others; some who need more carbohydrates, and some that fall in between.

Then there is the importance of balancing the ratio of your carbohydrate, protein, and fat intake. Nutritional experts all disagree on this topic – the main reason is that they're trying to find the perfect balance for all human kind. It doesn't exist. Each person is unique in their nutritional needs, yet what is common in our society is a negligence of basic nutritional knowledge. Therefore most of western society has no clue of what or what not to eat.

Two hot topics these days in nutrition are "metabolic typing" and "blood typing" for our specific food intake. I suspect that both are related in their importance. Basically, these nutritional programs are based on the fact that we are physiologically different depending upon our genetic make-up. I would like to recommend the following books, if you find this topic interesting:

DR. J'S RECOMMENDED BOOKS ON DIET:

The Metabolic Typing Diet: Customize Your Diet to Your Own Unique Body Chemistry
by William Linz Wolcott and Trish Fahey; Broadway Publishing
Pub. Date: January 2, 2002; ISBN-10: 0767905644

The Nutrition Solution: A Guide to Your Metabolic Type
by Harold J. Kristal, James M. Haig; North Atlantic Books
1st edition: December 9, 2002; ISBN-10: 1556434375

Eat Right 4 Your Type: The Individualized Diet Solution to Staying Healthy, Living Longer & Achieving Your Ideal Weight
by Peter J. D'Adamo and Catherine Whitney Publisher; Putnam Adult
Pub. Date: January 1, 1996; ISBN-10: 039914255X

The pH Balance Diet: Restore Your Acid-Alkaline Levels to Eliminate Toxins and Lose Weight by Bharti Vyas and Bharti Vyas, Ulysses Press
Pub. Date: July 6, 2007; ISBN-10: 1569756074

I don't recommend hopping on the latest diet fad. Every year there are new diet books that sell tens of thousands of copies. People are seeking that one miraculous diet that will allow for the most weight loss, usually at the expense of good nutritional intake. Because everyone has different metabolic types, the latest fad diet will not be right for an entire population of people. Remember that if you go *on* a diet, it means you must eventually get *off* it as well. Changing your health means changing your mentality about eating, not joining in on the latest diet craze. Begin a new consciousness of eating good food as a lifestyle choice. Change your "eating mindset" to begin adding more nutritious foods into your diet and make that important decision to take better care of yourself. Before you put a food or drink in your mouth ask yourself "Is this food improving my personal power and inner strength, or is it destroying my power and inner strength." Then make your decision on whether to eat it or not.

SUPPLEMENTATION

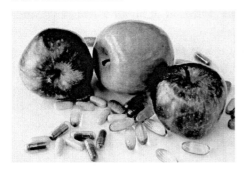

Most musicians, because of their schedule and life on the road, or working day jobs and performing at night, lack sufficient nutrients to ensure proper functioning of their bodies. Because western society has adopted the "fast food" mentality, we are sorely deficient of nutrients in our diet. This is why I highly recommend supplementation with *vitamins, minerals, essential fatty acids, and antioxidants.*

This doesn't mean that you have to become a pill junky. There are great products available that contain all of your needed nutrients in pill form, powder form, and in liquid form.

Liquid supplements have their pros and cons – as enzymes break down quickly in liquid form, and some experts think that the stomach acids will destroy most vitamins found in liquid supplements before they can be absorbed in the small intestine. Another point is that many liquid supplements are sold through multi-level marketing programs that boost up the price. But for those people who hate swallowing pills, they can achieve some added nutritional support through liquid vitamins.

Vitamin pills also have some drawbacks such as difficulty swallowing them. There are also cheaply produced pills, which will dissolve too quickly and be destroyed in the stomach, or they're not digested at all. These pills NEVER get absorbed and are excreted. What does that mean? You don't receive any benefit nutritionally and you can potentially waste a lot of money on them.

The manufacturing of vitamins is typically a man-made chemical process. Very few of the vitamins found in your favorite supplements actually come from nature. They are chemically manufactured in laboratories and produced for human consumption. I personally have a problem with ingesting man-made chemicals created in a lab. I would prefer to eat nature's source of vitamins: fruits and vegetables. So read your labels carefully and find out where the source of your vitamin supplements originate: The more natural and organic your source of vitamins and minerals, the better.

Good vitamin supplements are enterically coated, meaning they are created so that they do not break down too quickly in the stomach and they dissolve over time as they go through the small intestine. This allows the nutrients to be absorbed more efficiently and effectively.

The most important source for your nutrition is directly from the foods you eat. Enhance the amount of fruits and vegetables, particularly green leafy vegetables, in your diet. Spend more time in the grocery store investigating the vegetable aisle, and don't be afraid to invest in organic produce. You will reap the rewards of excellent nutritional care of yourself.

It takes tremendous work to ensure you and your family are receiving all the proper nutrients on a daily basis. For this reason, supplementation is usually a good idea to have an insurance policy that you and your family are receiving the necessary building blocks for cellular health. Trust me; this will be the financially cheapest and best insurance policy you will ever have.

There are a couple of supplements I recommend in my day-to-day practice as a doctor of chiropractic. First, I have finally found after twenty years in practice one of the finest sources of natural forms of vitamins, minerals, antioxidants, and greens; many from organic vegetable and fruit sources. The product is called **Greens First**. From their website, the product description reads:

> **Greens First** is a synergistic blend of 49 super foods, extracts and concentrates including super greens, organic fruits and vegetables, probiotics, soluble and insoluble fibers, herbs, spices, natural flavonoids and enzymes.
>
> © 2009 Wellness Watchers Global LLC
> (used by permission)

The use of this fantastic product is helpful at reducing the acidity of the body. The human body works best in a slightly alkaline environment. But, unfortunately, ingestion of many of today's foods and soft drinks, along with the caffeination of the world, leads to an out-of-balance, acidic body. This leads to weight gain, lowered immunity, an increased risk of cancer, poor organ function (particularly digestive problems), increased tendency towards musculoskeletal aches and pains, lowered energy levels, and a host of other symptoms and maladies.

The steady intake of greens, fruits, and vegetables help to reduce the acidity of the body, and restore the more natural alkalinity that the human body thrives upon. It has been shown that cancer cells do not replicate in alkaline environments, and in fact they die in very alkaline environments. That fact alone should be enough to encourage you to make a diet/lifestyle change immediately.

Every musician should be taking a greens super foods supplement on a daily basis. And of course, you now know that my choice is **Greens First**, which is produced by Wellness Watchers Global, LLC. If you are interested in learning more about this product, visit my personal website for this product: http://www.greensfirst.com/5699. You can order samples online and even set up your purchase online and have it shipped within a day or two directly to you. I encourage you to visit the website and discover the amazing benefits of a daily super foods intake. The best part is that it's really easy to make – just take an ounce of the powdered product, mix it with water, and you have an incredible mixture of ingredients that will undoubtedly take you to the next level of wellness! And it tastes great!

I also recommend supplementation with Omega-3 Essential Fatty Acids. You can find essential fatty acids in fish oils, flaxseed oil, and borage oil. The average western diet is very low in omega-three essential fatty acids, with an overabundance of omega-6 fatty acids. The body works at an optimum balance of the two forms of fatty acids. Our current fast food diet has immensely increased the proportions of Omega-6 to Omega-3's. When these go out of proportion the body lives in an inflammatory state, and any little irritation sets off inflammation and pain. This is not only true with muscular and skeletal conditions, but with internal organ malfunction such as asthma and inflammatory bowel disorders. Hormonal imbalances can also arise with an overabundance of Omega-6 fatty acids, and one of the most potent disturbances is mental irritability and depression.

Omega-3s are found primarily in cold-water fish like mackerel, salmon, and sardines. They promote a healthy mind, are naturally anti-inflammatory in nature, and promote healthy skin, balanced hormonal systems, and balanced body chemistry. You can also find excellent sources of Omega-3 fatty acids on my personal nutritional website http://www.greensfirst.com/5699. I am constantly amazed at the reports I get back from patients who see depression go away, inflammation and pain syndromes totally diminish, and mood swings depart as they get started on these supplements.

This company provides completely pure fish oil products that are cleaned of any impurities, especially heavy metals, mercury, environmental pollutants and pesticides. Many fish oils you find in drug stores and big-box stores are typically not purified. Be very careful about how much cheaply made fish oils you ingest – you could be poisoning yourself! My website explains the exact ingredients of all these products, their high level of pharmaceutical-grade production, and the excellence that the company stands by.

Although I truly believe in adding super foods and essential fatty acids to your daily regimen, natural sources of foods are always best. Some examples of antioxidant rich foods are blueberries, cranberries, acai berries, and many forms of beans such as red kidney beans and pinto beans. But some people enjoy knowing that they are insuring their nutritional intake whether it is through supplementation with vitamins or with super foods.

When you begin adding supplements to your diet, make sure you read the labels, because some brand name products actually contain lots of fillers and additives. I recommend avoiding generic brands found at your local drug store or at the large box stores. Invest in good vitamins for yourself if you feel you are not adequately receiving good nutrition in the food you are eating.

MAINTAINING BLOOD SUGAR LEVELS FOR OPTIMUM PERFORMANCE

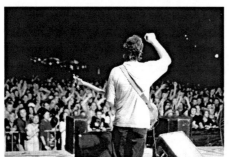

If you are on the road or even in your bedroom in a makeshift home studio, make sure that you are stocked up with fruits, vegetables, and protein sources such as cheese or nuts, for munching on during down time, especially for a brain recharge during an intense recording session.

Natural snacks, such as fruits and nuts, are much better choices than chips, dip, caffeine, and sugary candies or snacks, which are energy zappers that drastically impact your blood sugar and insulin levels. You may get a quick burst of energy after a sugary treat, but you will "crash and burn" about one to two hours afterwards because of the response of insulin to take the sugar out of your bloodstream.

Mixing a carbohydrate and protein together will provide a more constant blood sugar level and higher levels of brain function. Examples of these better choices are a banana with peanut butter, or having different forms of nuts available, or such excellent sources of proteins and carbohydrates like hummus or bean dip.

Nutritious food ingested every couple of hours will allow for a much more focused mind during recording sessions. The worst thing you can do is go more than three to four hours without food while recording, performing, and writing music. Your mind will not last because of lowered blood sugar levels due to the high demands of concentration necessary. This will lead to irritation, tendencies towards anger and frustration, poor playing ability, and wasted time and money.

If you are planning your day at the recording studio, think ahead and plan your eating schedule. Have snacks for every two hours between meals. Have a case of water ready to go! You will find that your abilities will be better, your skills will be well maintained, your voice will be clearer, and as you watch your buddies crash and burn from fatigue, you will be ready to go another few hours. Better yet, make sure your band members have the same snacks so everyone will enjoy a "fruitful" recording session and the band doesn't want to kill each other by the time the session is completed.

WATER INTAKE

Water is an essential nutrient that will determine how well your body functions. If you are dehydrated, your muscles are not going to respond as well to signals from the brain. A dehydrated muscle will injure more quickly. There is no standard amount of water that every person should take. Most nutritionists used to recommend six to eight glasses of water per day, but current science indicates that some people need less water, some more. This is similar to the metabolic types mentioned above. Your body has a range of water intake that it needs per day. The secret is figuring out how much water you personally need, and then maintaining that hydration level daily.

A good indicator of your hydration level is checking the color of your urine. If it is very light yellow to clear, then you are well hydrated. If it is very deep yellow in color, you are most likely dehydrated and should increase your water intake. (The color of your urine will change to a darker yellow if you are taking B vitamins, so it's best to not take vitamins while doing this test.)

Keep in mind that anything else you drink may interfere with your hydration levels. For example, caffeine containing drinks, such as coffee, teas, and colas will actually make your body urinate more, leading to higher levels of dehydration. Sugar laden sodas actually make you thirstier because of the increase of blood sugar levels after ingestion. There's about eight to ten teaspoons of sugar in soda. So drinking soda is not a substitute for drinking water. In fact, you'll need to increase your water intake if you are drinking sodas throughout the day.

Best yet – just get rid of soda from your diet. Diet soda is NOT an option because it also has poor properties. Every sugar substitute has been shown to cause health problems in adults. For example, Aspartame has been linked to tumors and blindness. Many studies have also shown that diet sodas actually caused increased levels of obesity due to the impact of the "fake" sugar on the human bloodstream. The body will actually feel increased hunger after drinking diet sodas due to the blood sugar changes that occur. Thus people eat more because of the hunger feeling.

Another key factor in hydration is alcohol intake. If you are a person who enjoys alcoholic beverages, just keep in mind that you should follow up for at least six hours afterward with increased water intake. Obviously, the amount of water depends upon your level of "enjoyment." If you wake up in the morning wondering how you got in the bed last night, then drink water all day long! Better yet, quit drinking alcohol!

If you are a vocalist, caffeine and alcohol are simply out of the question before a performance. Dehydration will impact the thin mucous layer that covers the vocal cords, making the mucous thick and sticky, which will dry out the cords and give you that "I need to clear my throat" feeling. I KNOW you know that feeling – you feel like you need to clear your throat every 30 seconds. Singers need a water maintenance plan to prevent this scenario and keep the cords healthy. Here it is: Plan on hydrating your body days before, during, and days after a vocal performance to reach for excellence in vocal artistry. It takes about an hour for the water you drink to be absorbed through the stomach into the cells of the body. So, if you think that taking in some water minutes before a vocal performance is helping your vocal cords, you're fooling yourself. You must plan hours in advance, hydrating yourself an hour or two before you sing, with fresh, spring water or purified water. Avoid tap water, as it has many impurities and added chemicals.

FIGHTING OBESITY

For those musicians whose waistlines are expanding at an alarming rate, measures must be taken NOW to begin the process of change. Weight gain is usually emotional in nature. Putting on the pounds can be a subconscious method of keeping people away from us, grounding us in times of extreme stress, or the result of depression or loss of self-worth. Sometimes, it is simply due to lack of knowledge in nutrition and decision-making in the types of food to eat and the type to avoid combined with a sedentary lifestyle.

If you find that you have put on quite a bit of weight over the years, then some self-investigation is needed to really understand why. Simply looking for diets to take some weight off is not always the answer. Because as you know, when you take off ten pounds, if the emotional stress has not been cleared, not only will you gain the ten pounds back, but you will probably gain an additional three or four.

Becoming your ideal weight begins in the mind. You have to reach a point where you finally say to yourself, "That's it, I have *had it* with this weight problem and I am willing to, learn, listen, understand, and do EVERYTHING I need to overcome it!"

This doesn't mean you need to starve yourself either. An understanding of nutrition is your first step. (Purchase one or more of the books recommended earlier in this book). Second is setting goals for yourself. (See the Wellness for the Mind section). Third, begin affirming to yourself that you deserve to look good, you are attractive, you are focused on becoming the ideal weight, and you do have the desire to exercise daily.

The actual physical part of losing the unnecessary weight really is very simple. All you have to do is burn off more calories per day than you take in. It's that simple! I have personally dealt with weight problems in my life, and I know first hand that to lose weight, I have to begin exercising at least five days per week, and I occasionally do two workouts a day. I watch what I eat carefully, usually having a protein shake for breakfast, salads for lunch, healthy snacks every couple of hours, and a well-balanced dinner. I definitely do not go hungry, and because of my higher metabolism from exercising so much, I burn off the food I eat, faster and more efficiently.

For those musicians who really struggle with weight loss, consider joining a support group like Weight Watchers®. This group uses sound principles to aid you in your quest to lose weight, become more fit, and optimize your health. The support group method works well, as you are encouraged to eat well and make better choices for your body.

We all know that obesity brings with it risks such as diabetes, atherosclerosis, heart disease, stroke, and many other ailments. An obese musician has other complicating factors as well, such as an increased tendency towards back pain because the instrument is further away from the body. Their overall energy levels tend to be less and fatigue will set in sooner while playing a gig or concert. With fatigue comes lowered mental clarity and decreased performance levels. Overall, the wellness-oriented musician will make the desired changes in his/her life to overcome a weight problem in order to reach optimal human function.

So make the decision to be healthier today. When you combine exercise with sensible eating habits and supplementation, the weight will melt off and your energy levels will skyrocket. Now let's move on to the next chapter where you'll learn how to maintain your body-instrument.

Chapter Four

WELLNESS FOR THE BODY – PART III – STRUCTURAL MAINTENANCE

WELLNESS OF THE BODY GOES BEYOND EXERCISE, diet, and nutrition. Being a Chiropractor, I feel it is my obligation to enlighten you on the benefits of my profession as well as lay some groundwork on how to allow your body to flow as a well-oiled machine. Let's begin with postural considerations.

"Watch your posture!" are everyone's favorite words to hear while playing an instrument. (Well maybe not.) These words are very important though, since your posture will determine the effectiveness of muscular movement and your ability to play a note efficiently and effectively. While I can't go over postural considerations for every instrument in this book, I can go over some basic knowledge that you should keep in the back of your mind while playing your instrument. First you need to learn about the structure that underlies your posture, and the impact it has on your health – the spine.

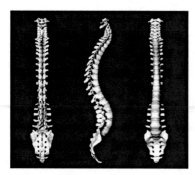

THE SPINE

The spine is made up of four curves, the cervical (neck) forward curve, the thoracic (mid back) backward curve, the lumbar (low back) forward curve, and the sacral (tailbone) backward curve.

Posture is all about keeping the spine in these curves while playing. Anything that changes the spinal curves for a prolonged period of time will cause strain upon both the spine and the nervous system that sits inside the spine.

For example, sitting with your head forward while playing guitar or piano will create strain in your neck muscles and will pull on the sensitive brain stem and spinal cord – especially if there already is decay in your spine. This can lead to nerve compression problems in your neck and radiating pain or tingling and numbness sensations in your arms and hands.

For musicians who are standing while playing, such as bassists/guitarists, keyboardists, stringed instrument players, percussionists, etc., watch how you are holding your body during these activities. I have seen guitarists who are in a constant state of forward flexion with the neck and upper body bent forward. Maintaining this posture over time will create a distorted, irritated spine and stressed nervous system. This may look "cool" on stage, but in twenty years, that guitarist is going to regret it when his spine is arthritic.

On the opposite end of the spectrum of postural disorders are the head-bangers. The constant repetitive forced forward and backward and side-to-side motion of the head causes tremendous wear and tear on the spine in the neck. I recently had a 20-year old head-banger lead rock guitarist in my office with complaints of arm pain and hand numbness. The x-rays showed degeneration of his spine – unusual for such an early age. Yet, he is constantly whiplashing himself by thrusting his head around continually while playing the guitar. I told him that if he wants to preserve what's left of his spine, his head-banging days 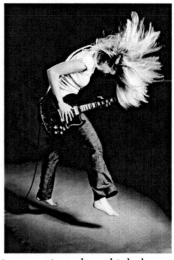 are over. That doesn't mean his music career is over, just the whiplash on-stage movements.

One of the most common symptoms I hear from musicians is tingling and numbness in the hands. Many times these symptoms are posture related. It is quite common to find nerve compression in the neck, shoulders, and arms because of bad postures. I like to videotape musicians to see how they're playing, because it tells me quite a bit about the reason for the symptoms. Some musicians have YouTube videos available or DVDs with their performances recorded. These offer tremendous insight into some of the reasons for the developing symptoms.

What these videos don't show is the stress the spine has been under for possibly years or decades BEFORE the video was taken. That's where a complete chiropractic exam and x-rays are needed to determine the extent of damage to your spine and nervous system. If you are interested in having your performance posture analyzed by me via YouTube or DVD, contact me via the email information at the end of this book.

To create a better posture, imagine as if you are being pulled upward by a cord that is attached to the top of your head. While you're sitting at the piano, or sitting in a chair strumming an acoustic guitar, that cord is tugging your neck upward, keeping your ears directly above your shoulders.

Obviously you are not going to be a stiff, unmoving person while playing. Maintain your artistic expression, but keep in mind that the head needs to wind up over those shoulders. The photo o the next page to the left shows a good, upright posture, while seated with a guitar. The photo on the right shows a typical posture that a new guitar player and even some seasoned players position themselves in as they play their guitar- bent forward looking at their hands or reading music. It's a back killer! Work on your posture now, and you can give you spine years of good health, and prevent many injuries.

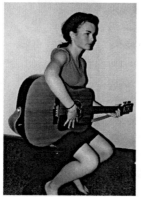 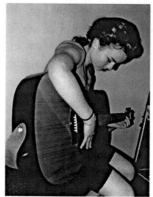

Some instrumentalists like to sit in a chair up against the chair-back. This is unadvisable because once you lock in your spine against the chair-back you cannot use inherent power of your torso muscles to play the instrument. (These muscles are known as the core.) This is especially important in string players, such as cello players, harp players, violinists and guitarists. You draw a considerable amount of energy for playing from the torso. If you doubt this, try playing a quick passage with your back locked against a chair. Then try it sitting upright and feel how this opens up your entire body to play the instrument with more speed and agility. I have personally tried to play piano in a standard chair, and not only is it uncomfortable as you try to lean forward to play the piano, it also does not allow for efficient playing or artistic expression.

Many orchestral musicians will use a small angled foam wedge on their seat to enhance their posture while playing the instrument. These wedges offer a small forward angle of about five degrees that slightly increases the lumbar curvature. Many instrumentalists note that this allows them to put more body movement into their playing, and keeps their backs from hurting after sitting for an hour or more. You can find these seat wedges at most instrument retailers or on the Internet.

Should you realize that attempting to sit up properly is really causing back pain and muscle spasms, you should consider an evaluation by a chiropractor to determine if there are spinal stresses that are irritating the sensitive nerve fibers. You may also be deconditioned with your postural muscles, and need rehabilitative training to strengthen them.

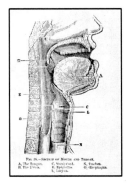

Fig. 39.—Section of Mouth and Throat.
A, The Tongue.   C, Vocal Cord.   N, Trachea.
B, The Uvula.   E, Epiglottis.   O, Œsophagus.
L, Larynx.

POSTURE AND THE VOCALIST

Your voice box, called the larynx, is directly impacted by your posture. A forward head posture, so common in today's culture, will force strain on the anterior neck muscles, and can even impact the nerves that supply life to the larynx and throat.

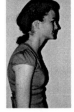

The forward head posture (shown on right) forces pressure upon the larynx and throat making them more susceptible to injury and chronic strain. This photo shows a poor, forward head posture (FHP).

The photo to the left shows a healthy posture, which will help to prevent symptoms such as hoarseness, chronic dry throat (no matter how much water you drink), nodules on the cords, or simply discomfort in the throat while singing, which can be caused by postural tensions and strain.

If you are experiencing any of these symptoms, observe your posture in a mirror or have someone snap a few photos of you. If your posture looks out of whack, you might consider bodywork, whether through a chiropractor, Feldenkrais® practitioner, or Alexander Technique practitioner to help relieve the underlying tensions creating the forward head posture. Your vocal abilities will be greatly improved once the posture issues have been remedied.

To finish out this chapter, I'd like to say that I don't expect you to perform stiffly. I understand that you need to move around and be in the moment of the performance, but you must remember to come back to a correct posture to free the body of unnecessary tension. Now let's move onto the next chapter to see if you are getting enough sleep.

Chapter Five

WELLNESS FOR THE BODY – PART IV – YOUR SLEEP HABITS

THE IMPORTANCE OF SLEEP

Sleep is an important aspect of health. If you have ever experienced a few days of sleep disruption, you know how much your body suffers. Your body is healing during the sleep hours. Your subconscious mind is releasing tensions from the day. Your cells are recuperating. Your body is preparing for another day ahead of usefulness and purpose.

If you are having difficulty sleeping, or are constantly waking up during sleep, it could mean your body is out of balance. Avoid caffeinated drinks for at least three hours before bedtime. Avoid alcoholic beverages before sleep as well, because alcohol changes the ability of the brain to go into deep sleep mode.

People who always wake up at the same time in the middle of the night may have organ system imbalances. Chiropractic and acupuncture techniques are available that can balance these organ systems and restore more natural sleep patterns.

Disrupted sleep also can point to mental stress, depression, or anxiety syndromes. *This doesn't mean that you should run to the medicine cabinet!* Drugs do nothing but mask the problem – if there is underlying stress that is affecting your sleep, then DEAL WITH IT! This might mean some counseling, talking to a friend, pastor, or mentor. Taking over the counter or prescription drugs will only create more problems as you deal with the side effects and the tendency towards addiction.

One added note: if you are a vocalist, and depend upon meds to aid in your sleep, you are really walking a thin line between imbalance and destruction of your voice. Medications used for sleep can dry out your throat, besides cause many other disorders. Here is a list of side effects from a popular sleep aid and pain reliever. This is directly from the site www.drugs.com:

Tylenol PM (acetaminophen and diphenhydramine) side effects. . .

Get emergency medical help if you have any of these signs of an allergic reaction: hives; difficulty breathing; swelling of your face, lips, tongue, or throat. Stop using this medication and call your doctor at once if you have any of these serious side effects:

- fast, pounding, or uneven heartbeats;
- confusion, hallucinations, unusual thoughts or behavior;
- severe dizziness, anxiety, restless feeling, or nervousness;
- urinating less than usual or not at all;
- easy bruising or bleeding, unusual weakness, fever, chills, body aches, flu symptoms; or
- nausea, stomach pain, low fever, loss of appetite, dark urine, clay-colored stools, jaundice (yellowing of the skin or eyes).
- Less serious side effects may include:
- dryness of the eyes, nose, and mouth;
- blurred vision;
- difficulty urinating;
- dizziness, drowsiness;
- problems with memory or concentration;
- ringing in your ears;
- restless or excitability (especially in children); or
- mild nausea, stomach pain, constipation.

After reading the above, do you honestly believe that taking this OTC drug or other similar medications will really aid in improving your "game?" You must be kidding yourself to think you are going to improve your singing ability or musicality by taking drugs to sleep at night. Find out the cause of your sleep disturbance and begin correcting the underlying imbalances that are causing the problem.

Over the counter and prescription medications are common causes of sleep disturbances. If you are experiencing problems sleeping, look first at what medications you are taking. Investigate their side effects on the Internet and discover if sleep disturbance is listed. Other medication side effects such as agitation, anxiety, depression, can also be an underlying cause for sleep loss. Alcohol use is another cause for sleep loss. Alcohol ingestion in the evening can change your body's ability to achieve deep REM sleep, and lead to abnormal sleeping and waking patterns that over time will wear you out. The last thing you want to do before a singing performance is overindulging in alcohol the night before. Not only will you sleep poorly, but you will also dry yourself out, have a hangover, and your voice will be very difficult to control due to dehydration.

There are some natural supplements that aid in sleep, such as valerian root, kava kava, and melatonin, but just like medications, these can become just another chemical you ingest on a daily basis to relax your brain. While these herbs do offer some benefit for sleep enhancement, the philosophy behind their usage is no different than chasing a drug in hope of a cure. If you are that wound up that you can't sleep, then become proactive and begin a relaxation program at least one hour before bedtime to begin winding down. This might mean some soft music, reading, prayer, meditation, or just quiet time without the kids pouncing on you.

Just a quick note here about a wonderful benefit of chiropractic care: one of the most common results I see from people receiving regular chiropractic spinal corrections is improved sleep habits. Many times, sleep disruption is caused by nervous system stress. The brain simply cannot allow the body to enter REM sleep because of all the abnormal signals barraging it from irritated pain receptors and body structural imbalances. Another reason people sleep better during the chiropractic program is because they typically decrease their medication intake as their body heals. Decreased meds means better health. Better health means better sleeping. So consider chiropractic as a resource for healing if you are currently dealing with sleep problems.

SLEEP AND CREATIVITY

What do you do when you are completely inspired, the creativity is flowing, and sleep is just getting in the way – yet you know you're tired? If you are on a creative binge, I would suggest going with it until you feel your mind has released all it has to offer. Trust me, that invisible power known as God will sustain you until the creativity has reached completion for that time period. Then sleep on it and wake up to refine it some more. But don't ignore sleep. Creativity is only good if the artist who created it stays alive to perform it! There are too many dead musicians who sacrificed their bodies for music. I wonder how many wonderful songs and melodies were we robbed of because the musician died before their time?

One final point about sleep is to consider the age of your mattress, and what style of mattress it is. In general, mattresses over ten years old are not sufficient to support your spine. Also, spring mattresses without the nice comfy foam padding on top tend to put too much pressure on your joints, compared to the new air mattresses and memory foam mattresses on the market. If you find yourself constantly tossing and turning while attempting to sleep, then your mattress may be to blame. Although mattresses can cost into the thousands of dollars, the impact they have on your health is very dramatic. Consider that you spend a third of your life asleep – what is it worth to sleep on a good mattress? It's a true investment in your health. And most good mattress stores have return policies to make sure you are happy with your investment.

One of the most common questions I get, as a chiropractor is, "hey doc, what's the best mattress?" It really depends upon your body type, size of your frame, health of your structure and many other factors. There is no "correct" mattress to buy, except for the one you lay on that gives you a great night's sleep. Time to go mattress shopping…

Now being on the road is a different story. You cannot control where you have to sleep when you are on a tour bus, in a car, hotel, plane, etc. But there are precautionary measures you can take, such as using the herbs mentioned in this chapter. Another thing that will help put you in the sleep state is a sleep mask that covers your eyes. It is a proven fact that light does indeed affect our ability to sleep well, so if you can cover up and use a sleep mask to block out as much light as possible; it will set you up for better sleep.

If you notice you are snoring, which will affect your sleep, you could try using snore trips, a mouth guard, or elevating your head with two pillows instead of one. All three will help to open the airways to assure that you receive the right amount of oxygen to help prevent snoring, and feed the body the oxygen it needs for a sound rest.

I've also heard many good recordings that help to put you to sleep, including a variety of sounds from rain and thunderstorms to dolphins or a train riding along on the tracks. If you can find a sound that is soothing to you, slap on a set of headphones, turn on the relaxing sound, and then cover your face and go to sleep.

Others use visuals such as counting sheep. In Jaime Vendera's book *Unleash Your Creative Mindset,* he presents a visualization that will help you drift off to sleep that combines the counting of numbers that are visualized in specific colors. If you make it through his visualization without falling asleep, I'll be surprised. Now that I've bored you to sleep, haha, let's move on to the next chapter where I will cover aspects of your environment that can affect you physically and how to deal with them.

Chapter Six

Wellness for the Body – Part V – Environmental Concerns

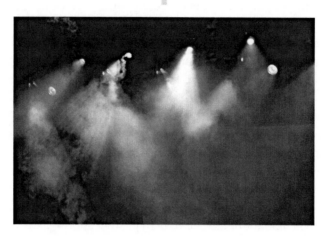

The Musician and Their Environment

The amateur or professional musician must become aware of their environment before they begin playing. "Environment" means such things as temperature where you will be playing, sun exposure, dry ice exposure, fog machine smoke, lighting, and noise exposure. A musician who investigates these aspects of his/her environment beforehand will be more capable of maintaining optimum health, while at the same time be prepared to perform at the highest level possible. Let us take a look at each of these different factors.

Ambient Room or Outdoor Air Temperature

Where will you be performing your gig? Is it in a concert hall with regulated air temperature? Or will it be in a cold, damp church on a winter morning? Make an attempt to visit your stage ahead of time to determine factors such as how you will need to dress, so you'll know whether you'll be subjected to a very cold environment, which will require more clothing or direct sunlight on a hot summer day. If you know ahead of time that you'll be performing in the heat, you wouldn't want to wear that flashy hot red polyester suit, because you'd suffer from heat exhaustion if you did.

Here are some great suggestions for dressing for the environment. If playing in cold environments, wear clothing that will keep your core body temperature maintained. If you are a singer, wear a scarf to keep the throat/neck warm. If your band or orchestra has standardized clothing, (aka "black") then consider wearing long underwear underneath your attire to keep you warm. Also, consider how the cold will affect your finger dexterity. Temperatures below 62° will lead to decreased dexterity and clumsiness. For cold weather performances, purchase a pair of gloves with the fingertips cut off, if playing your particular instrument allows this.

Maintaining hand warmth is critical to preventing repetitive strain injuries to the tendons and muscles. Besides that, your speed and dexterity are much better when your hand and fingers are warm.

If you are playing in warm environments, such as outdoors in the summer, remember to take with you at least two to four water bottles filled with spring or filtered water Take sips between every song if possible or at least every ten to fifteen minutes to maintain hydration. Even more important, it takes about one hour to hydrate your cells adequately, so begin drinking water at least one hour before the gig, not just during the gig. If you're only drinking water during the gig, it's good, but your body tissues may already be slightly dehydrated.

A part of hydration is allowing the skin to breathe in order to release toxins carried out by sweat. When performing, always wear clothing that can "breath" – allowing airflow to the skin, while allowing heat from the skin to escape. Avoid stuffy costumes and suits if at all possible. Have two towels handy - one to wipe off perspiration, and one that is dampened with cold water to wipe your head and face to help keep your body cool. Maintaining proper hydration days before the performance is just as important. Drink six to eight glasses of water daily in preparation for the hot climate.

THE JOYS OF THE STAGE!

Anyone involved in music production in stage shows or concert events knows that the combined effect of stage lighting, perspiration from performing, and sometimes anxiety or stage tensions, can make for a very hot environment to perform in. Preparation is the key. Unless this is your first performance in such conditions, you know that it is taxing – and therefore be prepared.

Extra towels, cool water, fans (if possible), and light, "breathable" clothing are important to protect your body against fatigue and exhaustion from the heat. I recently saw a photo of a rock artist who changed into his swim trunks because the stage was so hot from the heat of the venue, the lighting, and the ambient air temperature. It was actually good thinking on his part! Besides, it's rock n' roll – at least he had some clothes on, unlike some bands I know.

SUN EXPOSURE

Everyone knows that sun exposure increases the risk of burns and skin cancers. Musicians who are continually performing outdoor gigs throughout the summer months must take preventative measures to reduce the risk of any overexposure to the sun. Always use sunscreens with SPF 50 or greater. One application will keep you protected through a typical two-hour performance.

Wear sunglasses; make sure to wear sunglasses that block UV rays. It has been proven that sunglasses without an ultraviolet ray block can actually cause retinal damage to the eyes. Just because everything seems darker doesn't mean your eyes are being protected. Most sunglasses made today offer protection against UV rays. Don't skimp on your sunglasses if you're regularly performing outside. Wearing head protection is also important, particularly for those who are "follicularly-challenged." (better known as "bald"). A cap with a visor also helps to prevent glare from overhead lighting and from direct sunlight into your eyes. If that is rock-n-roll enough for you, tie a bandana around your head.

STAGE FOG

Large concert venues and theatrical venues enhance performances by using stage fog that reflects the lighting and offers more dramatic productions. Stage fog can be derived from a number of different substances, including glycerin, heated glycol alcohol (which is an ingredient in antifreeze) and fine particles of mineral oil, or liquid nitrogen. Many performers state that performing in the midst of stage fog irritates their throat and affects singing. If you are a singer, and have had a reaction to fog, tell the venue that you are allergic and you do NOT want stage fog during your performance. If fog is an important part of the show, request that the venue used a water-based fog.

Breathing in large amounts of carbon dioxide or glycol alcohol over a long period of time can affect your overall health. Many theatrical performers have complained, and even filed worker's compensation claims against production companies for voice and upper respiratory problems following long-term exposure to stage fog.

If you are involved in stage performances that include dry stage fog, consider the location where the fog will be blown from and attempt to position yourself and your equipment away from that location if possible. Talk with the production manager about pointing the fog machine away from the performers. In most cases, working together with the stage crew, production manager, and lighting director can provide the desired affects of the stage fog, while at the same time preserving the health of the musicians.

I often hear "fog" complaints from musicians who are situated in the "pit" just in front of and below the stage, particularly in theatrical productions. The fog will travel along the stage and then fall into the pit area, impacting the breathing abilities of the musicians. Contact the stage or production manager if this is the case, and seek a decrease in the amount and flow of the fog used. The flow can actually be controlled quite precisely with a knowledgeable person at the effects board.

NOISE EXPOSURE

Noise exposure can be very detrimental to the career of not only rock musicians, but every musician who is exposed to sounds louder than the normal speaking voice... Every musician must plan carefully on how they will handle the sounds on-stage or in the orchestra pit. Are you sitting directly behind a brass section that can reach over 100 decibels? Are you a bass player standing right next to a drummer? Consider the health of your ears. Prolonged exposure to loud noise WILL cause damage to the sensitive structures of the ears. Many types of earplugs exist for musicians that maintain adequate range of tones, while dampening the total decibels entering the ear. For comprehensive information on hearing issues, visit www.hearnet.net. This site offers many great articles about hearing loss and prevention issues.

One of the most popular ways of reducing on-stage volume is to use in-ear monitors. These reduce the necessity of on-stage monitors that increase overall volume. The musician or vocalist can receive the exact mix they desire, and at the exact sound level they desire. It's a wonderful way of preventing your lead guitarist from blasting you with a 110- decibel solo through the on-stage wedges. There are also earplugs specifically made for singers which can be found online.

LIGHTING

If you are reading music on-stage, will you be able to see the music with the lighting that's available? Or will you be straining every muscle in your face trying to see the music? Some music stands come with small lighting for this issue, but many do not. Again, planning ahead will prevent a great deal of discomfort, and will keep your eyes healthy. Will overhead lights or spotlights be directly in your eyes? Consider taking preventive action like sunglasses or visors to prevent being fatigued by glaring lights.

A musician who is serious about maintaining health will take a look at these factors as well as many others when preparing to perform. I can't repeat it enough; don't go into a performance without any prior knowledge of your playing environment. Knowing your environment is as important as the amount of practicing you have done over the past few years. Poor preparation can ruin your performance and even lead to health complaints down the line.

Here is a sample checklist that you can use when your band does a sound-check at a venue. Go through the following list, and consider your options for optimum health, reduced exposure to toxic elements, and injury prevention:

Sound Check Wellness Checklist

Overall environment considerations:
- Location of cords, pedals, platforms, stage configuration, tripping factors, edge of stage proximity to your location
- Location of sound outputs (monitors, other instruments, speaker arrays, amps)
- Ambient environment evaluation (sun exposure, room temperature, temperature of room)
- Location of fog machines
- Lighting design (light shining in eyes, ability to see instrument, necessity of eyewear, cap, etc.)
- Ability to read music (if you use sheet music during your performance) with current lighting design

Personal considerations:
- Clothing choices for environment
- Water availability
- Water intake prior to performance
- Ability to hear your vocals clearly to avoid vocal strain
- Sound levels of adjacent instruments and instruments running through your monitor (floor wedges or in-ears).
- Height of microphones – don't bend forward to sing! Keep the mic at a level that you slightly have to elevate your posture to reach it.
- For orchestral musicians – chair type, check adjustments to chair needed, room for instrument, location in pit, position among other players.

Bottom line; KNOW YOUR ENVIRONMENT! Let's move on.

Chapter Seven

WELLNESS FOR THE BODY – PART VI – INJURIES AND THEIR IMPACT ON YOUR CURRENT HEALTH

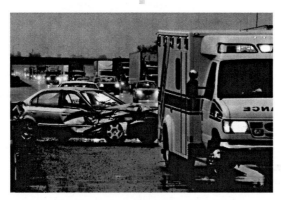

MANY PEOPLE SIMPLY NEGLECT THE FACT that your body accumulates stresses over a lifetime. Unless you take measures to erase them via methods such as chiropractic, massage therapy, or other bodywork techniques, your music career may be short-lived. Injuries such as previous car accidents, sports injuries, falls, serious traumas like broken bones and sprains/strains, repetitive traumas, and head injuries like concussions can lead to health problems later on in life that may affect your playing ability.

When considering why you may be experiencing health challenges, don't look just at what happened over the past month or year, but consider your life and what physical stress your body has endured. Have you suffered from poor posture throughout your life? Are you struggling with poor posture while playing your instrument? Chronic postural strain can lead to degenerative spinal conditions, nerve stress, and organ/system malfunction.

Previous car or motorcycle accidents can change the structure of the spinal curve in your neck. This accelerates the spinal decay and can lead to serious disorders such as tingling and numbness in the hands, cubital tunnel disorder, carpal tunnel syndrome, neck pain, back pain, TMJ disorders, and even internal problems like thyroid disorders and problems with your esophagus, vocal control issues and throat disorders.

For the musician who has lived a life enjoying competitive sports, you must consider previous injuries that you may have suffered, which could have impacted your structural function. These injuries can include sprains and strains, and/or injuries that involved impact with your body with any object, especially other people in contact sports. If you have ever suffered a force hard enough to create a concussion, then most likely there is some spinal trauma involved as well that was never detected before. Musicians rarely consider that previous injuries can have an impact on their current abilities. Yet they do, as your structure impacts your function. Any old injury that impacted your structure that never healed correctly will continue to haunt you unless you become proactive with a wellness approach to living.

On the other hand, if you have led a life completely free of injuries and have awesome posture and never had a strain of any muscle, then you're a rare and amazing human being! I doubt anyone can claim this though. Our bodies are amazing healing machines, but occasionally there are limitations in the healing process due to such problems as distortions in spinal structure and prolonged scar tissue formation. Also, chronic weaknesses of muscles can cause distortions of the skeletal system and the resulting aches and pains that are associated with them.

To find out where you stand with past health issues, consider consulting with a chiropractor, who will evaluate how your health history plays into your current health picture.

INTEGRATING CHIROPRACTIC INTO YOUR HEALTH REGIMEN

The cumulative effect of constant strains exerted upon the body from playing a musical instrument can lead to wear and tear on the muscles and joints. When you combine that with preexisting injuries and accidents, it is quite common for musicians to develop spinal and nervous system problems as a result. Abnormal tugging upon the spinal bones (vertebrae) due to overworked and tired muscles may lead to spinal misalignments (subluxations), nerve strain and pressure, increased tendency towards muscle spasm and loss of the normal range of motion in the joints.

Since chiropractors work with your nervous system – the primary controller of all bodily function – it is common for chiropractic practice members to experience improved overall health and wellness, not just muscular and joint pain reduction.

Chiropractic health care incorporates gentle realignments of the spinal and extremity joints to restore neurological balance within your body. The adjustments allow the natural flow of healing electrical impulses from the brain cells to the tissue cells via the nervous system. This restores health and well being to the body.

Spinal adjustments restore joint mobility, reduce muscle tension, restore nerve function to organs, tissues, and glands, improve brain function and mental clarity, increases immune function, and provide an overall sense of well-being. Hopefully, you can begin seeing how this important aspect of health care is necessary for the musician to achieve optimum wellness.

When you combine the improved wellness through chiropractic with the other recommendations for health enhancement you read in this book, you will be a powerhouse!

How Do I Find a Good Chiropractor?

I founded an international network of chiropractors who all have an avid interest of working with performing artists. To join my network, these chiropractors must have experience either as performing artists themselves, or have worked with numerous performing artists. Many of the chiropractors in my network work intimately with concert venues and theatrical venues, bringing chiropractic care on-site to musicians who are traveling through town. Also, all the chiropractors in my network understand the importance of subluxation correction and its impact of musicianship. For a referral in your area, go to www.musicianshealth.com and click on the "Find a Doctor" link to the Chiropractic Performing Arts Network.

Chapter Eight

WELLNESS FOR THE MIND

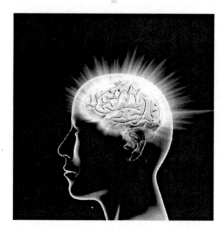

I think I should have no other mortal wants, if I could always have plenty of music. It seems to infuse strength into my limbs and ideas into my brain. Life seems to go on without effort, when I am filled with music.
GEORGE ELIOT (1819–1880)

WHAT YOU PUT IN IS WHAT YOU GET OUT

The mind is a powerful tool if used properly. The expression of your mind through body and spirit is dependent upon what you put in to it. It's similar to a computer. If you install corrupted data onto the hard drive, it will infect the entire hard drive and possibly destroy the output of the computer. Your brain is a computer. When you input negative information that is pessimistic, destructive, or depressing, you will reap a body and spirit that express these exact qualities, thus limiting your creative expression.

On the other hand, if you feed yourself with positive affirmations, goal setting, seek spiritual awareness, and treat your mind like a temple that cannot be destroyed, then your output will be beautiful. You will live a loving, caring lifestyle, seeking only the positive in life, and being a benefit for society, producing great music and being sought after for your talents. But all this takes a decision. The decision is what you should put in your mind. (If you want to read a great book on this approach, check out *Unleash Your Creative Mindset* by Jaime Vendera.) So let's take a look at what affects the wellness of mind, and then focus on how to avoid the negative and improve the positive.

TELEVISION

Most of what is on television is complete garbage. It will limit the creativity of your higher levels of brain function. The only hope for television is educational programs that expand our awareness and consciousness. If you grew up on MTV then your perception of reality is WARPED. If you decide to avoid the garbage channels, soap operas, cop shows, and violent cartoons, then you have taken one more step to control the wellness of your mind. How about the TV news? That's a quick way towards depression! Why would you want to input into your mind the latest rapes, murders, robberies, and political crossfires? I know many people addicted to TV news and their lives express the news they watch – lowered self-esteem, a negative view of mankind, a poor impression of a Divine Being, and in general, a lower vibrational level within their body.

Don't do this to yourself. Stay positive and let go of the negative. To improve your positive vibration, take a "news-fast". That's right – first go an entire day without reading ANY articles about the current news. Yes – that means on the Internet too – where a majority of people get their news these days. Then try it for two days and see the difference you feel mentally. You will feel more positive, upbeat, happy, and joyful, and most importantly, you didn't put any "garbage in."

BEING A "CONSCIOUS OBSERVER" WITHOUT ABSORBING NEGATIVITY

Social consciousness has been deeply impacted by music, and music has been deeply impacted by society. For example, think of the social impact of U2's *Sunday Bloody Sunday*, or Peter Gabriel's *Biko*. It is important for the socially conscious musician to understand current political and social trends. Writing music about them can bring tremendous change locally and globally.

Make sure you draw the line where negativity impacts your health, though. For example, you could become tremendously interested in the AIDS epidemic in Africa. You begin researching it more, reading up on the political actions being taken by various governments, and even become interested in the origin of AIDS, and the medical and natural ways of treating it. You may even write music about it. But don't go too far by internalizing stress because you become so absorbed in the topic that it begins eating away at your own health. Just remember to draw the line so your wellness and musicianship do not suffer.

Here's another example. You love to play "the blues." You become absorbed in the technique first, then you begin owning the lyrics, and then you BECOME the lyrics. Your life all of sudden is in turmoil, you can't keep a job, your spouse leaves you, you become sick. You have internalized the music that you enjoy. This is why it's called "the blues!" A healthy musician can play the blues with great proficiency and with great intention, but not let the subject matter eat at their own lives and health. The moral to the story is, as you become a great musician and vocalist you must feel the music and express it, but if you are singing musical lyrics that are potentially negative or depressing, don't be absorbed into them.

WHAT DO YOU DO BEFORE YOU FALL ASLEEP AT NIGHT?

One of the most important parts of the day for your mind is the hour before sleep. This is a critical time for impressions upon your subconscious mind. Do you watch the nighttime news before sleep? Do you realize that you are inputting negativity into your mind at the most impressionable time during the day? (You should, we just discussed this.) Why would you want to do that to yourself?

The hour before bedtime should be used as the time when your creativity flows. Read books that motivate you, read the Bible, write in a journal, write lyrics, pray, meditate, and the list goes on and on. This is your time to challenge your mind and create a positive influence for the next day. Do not miss this opportunity to create the life that you want, instead of dribbling in the leftovers of what other people are willing to give you.

THE MORNING ROUTINE

The next best time to challenge and positively influence your mind is immediately upon waking in the morning. Do you wake up and say "Good Morning, God!" Or do you say, "Oh God…it's morning!"?

Your attitude at the beginning of the day sets the standard for the rest of the day. A person seeking a wellness attitude for their mind will set aside at least 15 minutes, if not 30 - 60 minutes in the morning solely for the development of their mind, body, and spirit. Some of us in chiropractic call this the "Hour of Power."

A great morning routine that I have personally participated in begins about two hours before I need to leave for work. First, I thank God for another day of service to Him, and ask for His direction and guidance for the day ahead. I include some prayer time with this to further begin my spiritual journey for the day. Next, I exercise for at least a half-hour and during that exercise program, I state positive affirmations about myself, about my life, and about my purpose. This initial hour of self-mastery begins my day, so that I enter my chiropractic practice in the right state of mind ready for healing, communicating, and encouraging.

How do you start your day? Do you weaken your body chemistry with sugary cereals and coffee? Do you grumble and complain about getting up in the morning? (Well for the musician, it may be the afternoon!) Or do you appreciate another day of serving your life calling as a musician? Your attitude determines your day ahead. Remember this every morning, because you have the choice to create the direction your day will follow, both positively and negatively.

WHAT TYPE OF MUSIC ARE YOU LISTENING TO?

Again the same principle applies - garbage in, garbage out. If you are listening to music that is thought provoking, intuitive, and offers powerful and insightful lyrics, or music that is just simply beautiful, it will bring a positive neurological response to your mind, spirit and body. With this excellent, high vibration music entering your mind, your artistic expression both technically and musically will be enhanced.

On the other hand, if you listen to music that includes profane lyrics and is demeaning and harsh, your mind will respond by acting accordingly. Your musicality will also respond to this negative input by releasing garbage lyrics and fulfill the garbage-in, garbage-out philosophy. In essence, you can become the music you listen to.

If you want to enhance your musicality, carefully select your music choices. It may determine the level of professionalism that you achieve as a musician. Now I am not trying to convince you to change the style of music you play, but I just want to open your mind to the fact that music is a very emotionally charged, powerful life-affecting medium.

POSITIVE AFFIRMATIONS

An incredible way to change the way you perceive the world and change the way you act is to begin a daily regimen of saying positive affirmations to yourself. Life is so full of negativity with much of it is coming from ourselves; how we perceive our life, our bodies, and our future. Affirmations are exercises for the brain; a simple technique to counteract the mental negativity of the world. It's a way of telling yourself that you are okay, that your life is on purpose, and your work is fruitful and gifted.

Your subconscious mind is deeply carved by the time you reach just six years old. By this age, you know whether you are loved or not loved, whether you are happy or sad, whether you are sick or healthy, whether life is safe or fear-filled, whether your parents are loving or not, and hundreds of other distinctions.

Most people never consider the fact that they are carrying around the same notions about themselves that they have held on to since adolescence –whether they are correct or not! For example, some people think they are inherently bad because they were taught that idea as a child by their parents or their peers. You don't have to hold on to these old, incorrect notions! The first thing you need to do in this case is realize that what the mothers, fathers, teachers, and preachers told you about yourself may not be true! You are a beautiful creation – an awe-inspiring creation of God that has been given a life purpose. Never think of yourself less than that.

Begin picturing yourself as a child of God. Now that's a different notion than you've ever had! How can you be anything less than perfect if you were created by a divine being? You may have imperfections on the surface of various life abilities, but UNDER the surface - in your soul - you are a very perfect, beautiful, child of God.

Using affirmations can help you begin to understand that life is about positive creativity. I am hoping everyone reading this book has some sort of connection to believing in a supreme being. We make our own future by every day choices. It is much better to have faith, wake up with a positive attitude and see where it takes you. By hanging on to negativity, you'll never grow as an artist or a human being.

Affirmations should always stated in present tense, many times beginning with the words, "I am." Do not use negative phrases, like "I don't smoke." Change them to phrases with a positive reinforcement, like "I enjoy a life of clean air, clean lungs, and clean clothes by being free of smoking." In fact, from now on, never finish a negative sentence. Stop yourself and rephrase it immediately. Here are a number of examples for you to consider:

- I am a child of God
- I am a gifted musician
- I am a great singer
- My music reaches millions of people
- I am enjoying a life as a touring musician
- I eat healthy foods
- I am free of smoking
- I am wealthy in body, mind, and spirit
- I am filled with God's total abundance
- I am resourceful

- I am on time
- I am in touch with the Creator when writing music
- I enjoy great wealth because of my musical creations
- I am playing at Carnegie Hall
- I am reaching my desired weight of _____ pounds

That's a short list of affirmations. If you sit down and write in a journal, I guarantee you can write a list of at least a hundred positive things about yourself in an hour or less. Now the secret is to read these affirmations WITH EMOTION every day of your life, adding and subtracting them as you go along in your journey of self-enhancement. You do have the power to realize the beautiful person you were created and meant to be. Start right now by writing these powerful statements down on the space available to you on the following pages. Keep this book with you and read these affirmations daily.

MY AFFIRMATIONS
Write affirmations about yourself on the lines below

_____

_____

_____

_____

_____

_____

_____

_____

_____

_____

_____

_____

_____

THE SUCCESS JOURNAL

Another powerful wellness technique for the mind is journaling. It's time to begin a "success journal." In this journal, write down every successful event that happens during your day. This is usually done before bedtime. Write down lyrics that suddenly pop in your mind. Write down goals for yourself (more on that later). Write down people you met and 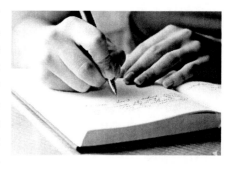 their impact on your life – or people you want to meet!

Writing down these facts will begin changing your subconscious and your conscious mind to again show you how really awesome you are. What does a success journal entry look like? Here's an example: "Met with record label rep today and the deal is on! Had tremendous inspiration on the lyrics I've been struggling with. Exercised for 30 minutes today!" You get the idea – now get to work!

Your local bookstore will carry a wide variety of journals – basically books filled with lined or unlined empty pages just waiting for your wisdom fill them with new understanding and creativity.

SETTING GOALS

Your mind needs a target. If you want to take a vacation and you get in the car without a destination in mind, this would be the height of stupidity. Yet many musicians live life this way. How about showing up at the airport without any flight reservations and then ask, "Where should I go?" This is what life would 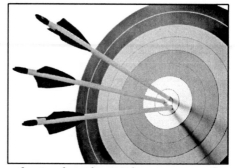 be like without setting personal and professional goals. Without a target for your brain, you will receive the leftovers of others who know where they want to go and what they want to achieve. Without any goals and dreams, your life meanders through any pathway that comes along, bringing you to destinations that may or may not hold beneficial outcomes.

Now just because you set goals doesn't mean that life will be glorious and you will attain them with absolutely no struggles. In fact, I can guarantee you that the more goals you set, the more struggles you will need to overcome.

More goals mean more failures and more learning experiences. Nature will test your strengths and weaknesses. Nature will test your willingness to overcome obstacles. But if you hold the course, overcome the tests, and get past the inevitable "failures," you will achieve those goals you set out for. In fact, quit thinking of them as failures, and begin viewing them as learning experiences.

Every musician who reaches the top of the charts will tell you how driven they were to achieve that level of success. They set goals, even as a child, on how successful they would become. They knew the outcome before it occurred. Some actually visualized in their mind their success, years before it happened. Are you doing this today? Can you see yourself on stage in front of thousands of screaming, adoring fans? That's goal setting.

There's nothing wrong about setting goals for yourself, as long as they are goals that will not just benefit you, but benefit humanity as well. If your goals are selfish – guess what, you might achieve them, but will feel incredibly unfulfilled once achieved. Short term gratification may be fun temporarily, but in the long term it is terribly unsatisfying as we seek our purpose in life. For example, you may have a goal to have a red Porsche Carrera convertible in five years. This is what I would call a "selfish" goal. Anyone with good credit can buy a Porsche and then be $80,000 in debt. That's not a goal, that's poor financial planning and is ego-driven.

Consider this goal as a healthier alternative: "By (enter date here), I will have played my music before an audience of 15,000, and will enjoy the tremendous return of wealth due to ticket, merchandise sales, and royalties. The music performed inspired everyone and surpassed the audiences' expectations for level of performance. As a result of providing positive, uplifting music to humanity and using my God-given gifts, I will be able to attain one of my life's personal goals; a beautiful red Porsche 911 Carrera, paid in cash." This goal is much different because there is an exchange that takes place in return for your hard work and musicianship that blessed many. You can go further with this goal writing by adding how much money you want to attain and when you will achieve it by – and more importantly what good you will do for mankind through your acquisition of money.

Goals also have different maturation rates. I like to think of them sitting in an incubator over time. As you go through life and work towards your goals, they will be completed at the perfect time and in the perfect place. That's why you should have short-term goals (weeks to months), medium-term goals (months to years), and long-term goals, (5, 10, 20 year goals).

There are different forms of goals. These are called the "Six Ps."

Purpose: This is your mission statement. Why were you put on this planet? What difference are you going to make to mankind by being alive? What legacy will you leave?

Personal Goals: These could be such things as exercise goals, attaining a healthier weight, changing habits. What people do you want to meet? What things do you want to accomplish?

Professional Goals: When do you want to sign your first record deal? Or, when do you want your first gold record? How about platinum record? Simpler goals could be writing your first song, or learning to play a new instrument.

People Goals: Who would you like to work with, or be closer with? Who are some personal heroes you want to meet? Who would you like to *get away from?*

Prosperity Goals: How much money do you want to make and save? What is your financial master plan? Decide on becoming more competent in where you are financially sound. Learn to set up a budget. Make a goal of restoring and maintaining good credit.

Play Goals: Don't forget the fun stuff – vacations, culture, entertainment, jewelry, clothing, donating time, etc.

In the next few pages, I'll present you with a place to write down answers to your goals (Six P's). After you do this, number the goals in order of importance. Work on goals that are in place to develop your personal growth. These must always occur first for you to do the actions to have what you want in life.

Write your goals in more than one place. Don't just write them in this book, and then close the pages. Keep them in your office, home, and in your music studio. The more you look at them, the more they are likely to happen, because your subconscious will be inspired to see each goal completed.

Each goal you write should have a date of completion. Any time you complete a goal, write a big "SUCCESS" after it. This empowers you to complete more goals.

Finally, goal setting doesn't have to be only for wondrous, lofty concepts or for costly material items. A simple personal goal can be "I'm getting up a half-hour earlier, five days per week, to allow time for exercise." You'll find it easier to accomplish these smaller goals, and they help you realize that you can direct your mind to complete goals. Once this happens, your life blossoms and you become empowered.

For more information about goal setting, I recommend books, videos, and CDs by Mark Victor Hansen — co-author of the *Chicken Soup for the Soul* series. His web site is www.markvictorhansen.com. Also, check out the following books:

DR. J'S RECOMMENDED BOOKS ON GOAL SETTING:

Make Success Measurable!: A Mindbook-Workbook for Setting Goals and Taking Action by Douglas K. Smith Wiley
1 edition: February 26, 1999; ISBN-10: 0471295590

The Complete Idiot's Guide to Reaching Your Goals
ISBN-10: 002862114X

(All recommended books can be quickly found by visiting my website www.musicianshealth.com and clicking on the "recommended books" tab)

Some examples of goal setting:

TARGET DATE	GOAL	ACHIEVED?
9/1/	Run 5 K!	
10/15	Complete songwriting for CD	
11/1	Send songs to indie producer	
11/30	Have vacation next June paid for!	
5/1	Date night with wife once per week begins	
7/1	Have $10,000 saved in savings account	

These are some quick examples — I recommend elaborating and being very detailed about your goals. Don't forget to place a number in front of the most important goals you want to achieve. Your brain needs a target. GO FOR IT!

MY GOALS

PURPOSE:

_____

_____

_____

_____

PERSONAL:

_____

_____

_____

_____

PROFESSIONAL:

_____

_____

_____

_____

PEOPLE:

_____

_____

_____

_____

PROSPERITY:

_____

_____

_____

_____

PLAY:

_____

_____

_____

_____

FINANCIAL WELLNESS

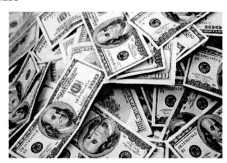

Annual income twenty pounds, annual expenditure nineteen six, result happiness.
Annual income twenty pounds, annual expenditure twenty pound ought and six,
result misery.
CHARLES DICKENS (1812–1870), David Copperfield, 1849

A large portion of our society is heavily in debt. Debt is a sure-fire way to destroy your wellness. If you are currently in debt, you **must** begin a strategy to get out of it. You cannot reach optimal wellness as a musician with tons of debt. Debt is like a 100-pound weight around your shoulders. It will bring you down, literally, in all aspects of health, including physically, spiritually, and mentally. There are many books on the topic of getting out of debt. Here is a quick list of the many books available to you:

DR. J'S RECOMMENDED BOOKS ON GETTING OUT OF DEBT:

*How to Get Out of Debt, Stay Out of Debt, and Live Prosperously: *(Based on the Proven Principles and Techniques of Debtors Anonymous)* by Jerrold Mundis; Bantam Books,
Pub. Date: Jan 1, 2003; ISBN-10: 0553382020

The Total Money Makeover: A Proven Plan for Financial Fitness by
Dave Ramsey Publisher: Thomas Nelson;
2 edition: February 6, 2007; ISBN-10: 0785289089

Your Money Counts by Jr., Howard L. Dayton; Tyndale House
Publishers
Pub Date: Mar 3, 1997; ISBN-10: 0842385924

*(All recommended books can be quickly found by visiting my website
www.musicianshealth.com and clicking on the "recommended books" tab)*

I recommend you begin reading more on this subject if you find yourself constantly trying to pay off credit cards, are behind all the time on payments, and especially if you find yourself near bankruptcy. There are also non-profit agencies that can help you overcome severe debt problems by working with your creditors and developing a repayment schedule.

Many musicians struggle early in their careers financially, and some struggle their entire careers, usually working one or two other jobs to help support their music. I know, as a musician, you need gear. But instead of feeling like you need to buy everything brand spanking new, check out eBay or Craigslist for used equipment. Remember, it's the musician that makes the instrument, not the other way around, so you don't need to go in debt for a $2000.00 guitar, thinking it'll turn you into a superstar. Practice and a positive attitude will turn you into a superstar! So, use your money wisely and you will begin a trend of saving and prosperity that will continue with you as you become a more established musician.

"Where do I begin to make changes to my financial crises?" The following keys to financial wellness are a great starting point to help you regain control of your financial life:

1) Save 10% of everything you make. Pay yourself first! That doesn't mean keep 10% and blow it on booze or material items. This money is NOT to be used for any purpose but for investments. Invest this money into financial vehicles that will make even more money for you by the wonderful concept called "interest." By the way, a simple bank account, making one or two percent interest is actually losing money for you. Seek other investment strategies such as mutual funds to enhance your financial wellness. Seek council on these matters with a financial consultant.

2) Tithe 10% of your income to your church or give the 10% to organizations that meet the needs of human beings spiritually, emotionally, and physically.

3) Use the rest of your money to pay bills, live on, and if there is excess still left over, continue to save it. And enjoy life!

4) DO NOT BUY ANY ITEMS FOR DAILY LIVING UNLESS YOU CAN PAY FOR IT WITH CASH! Do not put yourself in debilitating debt because of desires for a 50-inch TV, and boutique amplifier, or a fancy sports car. One of the biggest issues in financial success is self-control. Don't forget eBay.

5) Destroy all your credit cards except for one to be used for such things as booking rental cars, flights, etc. (as long as you pay off that card immediately without lapsing into debt.)

6) Use debit cards from your bank for purchases when you don't have cash. This way money comes directly out of your bank account for the purchase.

7) Look at your monthly expenses and cut out what you don't need. Do you REALLY need a home phone and cell phone? Do you have to have the premium television package? Can you turn off the lights during the day to save $10.00 a month on electric? Do you REALLY need to smoke two packs of cigarettes and day? (Which, by the way, is a several hundred dollar a month habit.)

For more information on these topics, I recommend:

DR. J'S RECOMMENDED BOOKS ON PROSPERITY:

The Richest Man in Babylon by George S. Clason: BN Publishing
Pub. Date: December 17, 2008; ISBN-10: 1607960664

The One-Minute Millionaire: The Enlightened Way to Wealth by
Mark Victor Hansen and Robert G. Allen; Three Rivers Press
Reprint edition: August 4, 2009; ISBN-10: 0307451569

Dynamic Laws of Prosperity by Catherine Ponder: bnpublishing.com
Pub. Date: September 12, 2008; ISBN-10: 9562912469

*(All recommended books can be quickly found by visiting my website
www.musicianshealth.com and clicking on the "recommended books" tab)*

These books will retrain your mind to begin thinking prosperously, and understand that money impacts your life both mentally and spiritually.

For those of you who are really struggling with the whole concept of making money, or maybe don't feel worthy of making money, I would recommend the book *Rich Dad, Poor Dad* by Robert T. Kiyosaki. This book investigates how we learn about handling and making money early on in our lives from parental influences. You *can* change the way to think about money. Money in and of itself' is not bad. What is bad is when you become greedy and seek more and more money for yourself without any benefit to society as a whole. As the Bible states, "The LOVE of money is the root of all evil."

Many people have misinterpreted this statement that money is bad. The passage goes on to state in the Bible in 1 Timothy 6:10, "Some people, eager for money, have wandered from the faith and pierced themselves with many griefs." So the warning in this biblical passage is to not allow the desire or greed for money cause you to stray from your faith. In other words don't allow money to become your god. Put the real God first in your life, and all other endeavors below that in their proper perspective.

In *The One Minute Millionaire*, Robert Allen speaks of "Enlightened Millionaires," who have tremendous fun making money because of excellent products and services they offer, and in return give 10% of the earnings back to worthy charities, churches, and organizations to make a difference in our world. Money can be a very powerful tool if used wisely.

What do you do with your money? Do you squander it as soon as it hits your wallet? Do you hoard it and never let a penny go to serve others? Or do you use is wisely to serve, to bless others, and to support your family? It is time to really learn about the impact money has upon your life. Purchase some of the recommended books listed in this chapter, and begin a new "chapter" in your life in regards to financial freedom and financial wisdom.

Alas we have reached the final phase of Mind, Body & Spirit. In the next chapter I will show you how discover a spiritual side of yourself so that you are completely healthy, wealthy, creative and successful.

Chapter Nine

SPIRITUAL WELLNESS: WE ARE ALL SPIRITUAL BEINGS

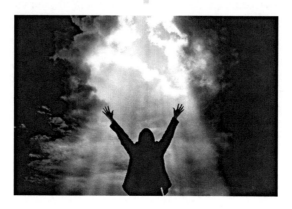

Think of yourself as an incandescent power, illuminated and perhaps forever talked to by God and his messengers.
BRENDA UELAND

For the most part, human beings are constantly seeking a more spiritually fulfilled life. It is my view that humans are in actuality, spiritual beings placed temporarily in the physical coats we call bodies. We are not, as some would think, physical beings seeking some type of spiritual life only when it is comfortable or convenient.

I believe in a higher spiritual being, a creator, a loving God. If you are hesitant about belief in a higher being, or simply do not believe in a higher being, I ask that you read through this chapter with an open mind. My personal faith in God has been instrumental in my success in life – in family, business, relationships, physically, mentally, and spiritually, so I wanted to share every part of that success with you. It never hurts to hear another person's views about spirituality. That's how we grow.

If you want to grow spiritually and possibly make decisions that will change your entire life and your viewpoint of life, then read on. If you would like to tap into the intelligence that exists in our creator to enhance your songwriting skills and your performance, then this chapter will help you understand how. If you are currently seeking a higher level of spirituality but do not consider yourself a very religious person or lack knowledge on the subject, then I encourage you to read on. This message may give you some answers to questions that have been crossing your mind lately.

CAN MUSIC IMPACT YOU SPIRITUALLY?
CAN YOU IMPACT OTHERS SPIRITUALLY WITH YOUR MUSIC?

Have you ever listened to a performer that touched your heart so deeply that you could not stop crying? That is an example of a complete circle of the mind/body/spirit reaction. Anyone who has experience of sitting in a church and being deeply impacted by a soloist pouring their heart out to God will tell you that spirituality is an integral part of music. It's important to understand that the music itself does not have to be in the spiritual music genre to touch you spiritually. For example, if you listen to a canon by Bach, your spirit is impacted by every note performed. In the same line of thinking, the music you write on a page has the potential of deeply impacting someone spiritually.

GOOD VS. EVIL

Spirituality comes in two forms though. In all things, opposites exist. There is cold and hot. There are both valleys and mountaintops. There is rich and poor. There is elation and depression. There are also good spiritual beings and bad spiritual beings, which are taught in most world religions. Some people equate goodness to the brilliance of light (God-like) versus absolute darkness (Satan-like). Consider it as you may, both ends of the spectrum exist. Understanding this important concept has a tremendous impact on your music and your songwriting.

WHERE DOES YOUR INSPIRATION COME FROM?

Just as the light of the all-powerful God can infiltrate our music and our life, we can also be influenced by the evil-natured darkness. (Entire portions of the music industry are based upon this fact, profiting off of people's lives to fill them with dark music). Start seriously investigating the lyrics you've written lately or the music you have listened to. Is the music lifting people up and enhancing lives, creating positive social change and exposing the unjust? Or, are the lyrics dark, profane, and cynical and attempting to influence others into disturbing rituals, demeaning to races or genders, or lead to activities that destroy life such as encouraging drug use and promiscuous sexuality?

Think of it this way; everything is vibration, thus we are vibration, life is vibration, music is vibration. Look at a guitar string vibrating. Every vibration has an impact on your body and you can "tune" to it. Would you rather be positively or negatively tuned?

Music that enhances life and builds people up is an example of God-inspired (positive) music. Music that has the ability to destroy is an example of negative, dark music. Guess what, they are *both* spiritual in nature! But they have opposite reactions to both the listener and the writer. What you write will impact people possibly for generations to come. The responsibility you have in your writing is awesome. Don't ever underestimate your potential to impact lives – whether it is positively or negatively.

This is not to say that all music must be happy, upbeat, and cheerful. Some of the most profound and impactful music ever written is by artists going through tremendous life hardships, and the music tells the story of their angst. We listen and relate to it because many of us have been there ourselves, or are going through the same ordeal when you are listening to the song. Yet, even though the music may be sad and tug at our hearts, it does not lead us into destruction. That's the big difference. When the artist has an *intent whether willfully, spiritually, or subconsciously* in writing music to negatively influence others, they are living and expressing their life in darkness or as the analogy above states, living in a negative vibratory state.

What is your health worth? Are you willing to listen to music that destroys you from the very essence of your soul? If you are a writer, think about what you are writing. Will it impact human lives in a positive way? Are you making a positive difference in the world? You can express life's challenges through your music without influencing your listener to re-enact that negative experience.

One final word on this subject: if you are creating music that is destructive to the human soul, and are profiting off of that music, you are stealing and cheating your way through life at the expense of people's souls and their health, and their family's health. YOU are responsible for YOUR actions. And YOUR actions impact OTHERS' actions. I pray that you will consider the impact your music has upon humanity, and decide to impact the world in a constructive matter through your music.

THAT "SPARK" OF CREATIVITY

We must accept that this creative pulse within us is God's creative pulse itself.
JOSEPH CHILTON PEARCE

As we are composing music, we often get that incredible spark of creativity that brings tremendous insight, knowledge, or just a rhyme that has eluded us for hours. Have you ever thought about where that spark came from? This is where our spirituality and our mind interplay together with a divine being. Our mind contains our past and current experiences. When we combine this limited educated knowledge with an omniscient God via our spirituality, we receive inspiration that sometimes seems incomprehensible. With this understanding, you as a musician can begin learning how to tap into that incredible spiritual source that will allow your creativity to flow and your spiritual wellness to reach optimum levels.

Be very careful of your intent with your music, because that spark of creativity will come – but where is it coming from? Because your music can impact countless lives, you are on the spiritual front lines. The information you read below can help you strengthen your spirituality and better yet, accept the wonderful love that God has ready for you, if you are willing to open your heart and accept it.

GIVING THANKS

God has two dwellings: one in heaven, and the other in a meek and thankful heart.
IZAAK WALTON (1593–1683)

An important step towards spiritually inspired music is to give thanks for all things – even the struggles. For with every struggle, there is spiritual growth, character building, perseverance, hope, and a solution. When you reach deep down within your heart and show total love, you cannot help but begin rejoicing and thanking every day of your life.

So begin the process right now! Reach down inside yourself and begin offering thanks for everything in your life. If you have food on your table tonight, give thanks. If you have a place to sleep tonight, give thanks. If you have a guitar that is playable, give thanks. These "thanks" go to our creator, for without Him we are just dust.

If you begin thanking every day, and live your life in "thanking mode" you will see that spiritual wellness permeating not just your own soul, but also those who you come in contact with. Make an effort to send three thank you notes per week to anyone you have come in contact with that has benefited your life or the lives of others. Send a thank you note to the mechanic who changed your car oil last week. Send a thank you note to your parents, even if they weren't the absolute best parents in the world. Send a thank you note to a fellow music buddy who you enjoy rehearsing or performing with. Become a person of thanks. If dropping notes in the mail isn't your style, send them a "thank you" email. Our society today has seemingly forgotten the art of thankfulness as it seeks constant self-gratification.

Thankfulness puts others before your own self; it creates a heart to see others be lifted up. It is a very healthy lifestyle. If you consistently do this action over a period of a year or more, you will develop a reputation as a loving individual, who puts others before themselves. That is an incredibly desirable reputation that is admired by everyone. Create a legacy for yourself and for your family of living, loving, serving, and thanking.

WHAT'S YOUR SPIRITUAL PURPOSE?

Why were you placed on this planet as a musician? What is your calling? What are you doing that is honoring the creator that gave you life and the gift of music? These are all deep questions that take days, and sometime months or years to figure out. If you want your music to impact lives, then you have to begin asking yourself these important questions. When you begin understanding your purpose in life and how it pertains to your musical gifts, there will be a renewed spark that changes your creativity, passion, and love of music, and beyond that, your love and joy of life itself.

If you write music *just to make money*, the excitement of writing and performing music can quickly come to an end when either:

1) You become very successful and you have achieved opulent wealth, or
2) You are broke and your music does not support your lifestyle.

Either end of the spectrum will destroy your happiness and inner joy if the reason is solely to make money. The secret ingredient is the inner passion that drives you. Passion leads people to write their deepest feelings and beliefs into song. When you reach this point of creativity and depth, it doesn't matter whether money is coming in or not, because the music must be written no matter what the consequences or rewards. Money will come when people are attracted to your deep passion for your music, its quality, and its impactful message.

I know that as a struggling artist, your finances must be a concern for a healthy life balance. That is why so many musicians have "real jobs" to provide income for themselves and their families as they pursue their music career. There are the rare few who make a full living off of producing, selling, and performing music. If you are one of these, give thanks for that tremendous blessing you have received. If you are not one of these, then continue striving to pursue your dream, and find a great passion-filled career that supplements your other passion- music.

I pay no attention whatever to anybody's praise or blame. I simply follow my own feelings.
WOLFGANG AMADEUS MOZART (1756–1791)

Is music truly your spiritual purpose? What happens if after deep introspection you begin realizing that playing music may not be your life's calling? Congratulations! You have made a major distinction in your life, and you now can set a path for your future. Music will always be there, and you can always play music whether it is in a local café, at your church, or in a garage with friends. But if your true calling to benefit mankind is to impact people through other avenues, then go deep within your soul, seek out the direction of life that your heart is set upon, set your goals, write out an action plan, and GO FOR IT!

Here are some questions that you need to ask yourself on a regular basis.

1. "If I had no monetary limitations and were financially free, what would I do with my life?" (This will allow you to tap into your true calling without limiting thoughts about money.) Write your answers below.

_____

_____

_____

_____

"If I believe that I was created by a loving God who inspired me with great talents and gifts to be used for the good of humanity, what would I be doing differently in my life?" "What would I be doing the same?"

_____

_____

_____

_____

3. "In the deepest recesses of my heart, I feel compelled to
    _____ to make
    this world a better place.

If you answered- "play music" to these questions, then you are on track for your future. But if you did not provide that answer, or if you don't know the answers to these soul-searching questions, then further investigation and self-discovery are needed.

How do you find your calling? First off, you must become in touch with your heart and through your heart, tap into the source of creation, which is God. If you have erected four-foot thick, stone walls around you to protect you from others, from God, and from your own heart, then those walls are going to have to begin tumbling down. Sincerely ask God why you were placed here. Ask Him who the real _____ (insert your name here) is.

Prayer is a powerful way to realize your reason for being. You don't have to pray as if God is one billion miles away from you either. He is right next to you, listening intently to you, with a desire of close relationship with you. Speak to Him, ask Him for direction; allow Him to speak to your heart. For more information on this subject, check out the following book:

DR. J'S RECOMMENDED BOOKS ON FINDING YOUR PURPOSE:

The Purpose Driven® Life: What on Earth Am I Here For?
by Rick Warren; Zondervan
Pub. Date: March 13, 2007; ISBN-10: 0310276993

HAVING FAITH

Now faith is being sure of what we hoped for and certain of what we do not see.
HEBREWS 11:1

What do you put your faith in? Is it your money? Is it God? Is it in your family? Is it totally in yourself and your abilities? Or, do you have faith in absolutely nothing? Faith is one of the driving factors in our lives. Faith is a uniquely human attribute, offering a reason for living. Life without faith is creates a miserable existence of self-absorption, dependencies, inner sadness, and lack of drive. Life with a strong faith compels a person into action, releases ambition, creates endurance, and builds character.

You must have faith to write that first song. You must have faith to take the stage for the first (or even hundredth) time. You must have faith to make a change in the world. Therefore, faith is an important part of overall spiritual wellness. You need faith to be a spiritually driven musician. Higher levels of faith bring higher levels of spiritual wellness and higher levels of certainty and trust.

On the other hand, you cannot grow spiritually with little faith in a loving creator, or little faith in others or in yourself.

> "But faith isn't always that easy, even for people who desperately want it. Some people hunger for spiritual certainty, yet something hinders them from experiencing it. They wish they could taste that kind of freedom, but obstacles block their paths. Objections pester them. Doubts mock them. Their hearts want to soar to God; their intellects keep them securely tied down."
> —*The Case for Faith*, **LEE STROBEL, P. 8**

Is your quest for spiritual enlightenment being blocked by a difficulty in having faith in something that cannot be seen? Many people have enhanced their faith in a creator (God) by simply looking at nature. Many steadfast atheistic scientists have changed their views on God by simply investigating the simplest microscopic organisms in detail. Seeing the complexity of nature in even the simplest of organisms, points to a divine creator.

> *"Faith is about a choice, a step of the will, a decision to want to know God personally. It's saying 'I believe-please help my unbelief!'"*
> —*The Case for Faith*, **LEE STROBEL, P. 255**

> *For those who struggle with questions about faith in God, I highly recommend the book that I quoted twice here, Lee Strobel's* The Case for Faith.
> **(ZONDERVAN, 2000)**

FINDING GOD
Warning: The following information may radically change your life and will fill your heart with the love of God. Expect a miracle to happen!

If this whole idea of asking God for help, prayer, or spirituality is new or foreign to you, then I would like to offer you the following clues as to how to find God, and how to ask Him into your life:

1) Become humble: realize the world does not revolve around you and your desires for greatness. If you believe in a God, then humble yourself before Him and ask for His mercy and grace, and that you will be filled in His promise for greatness in your life. Even if you don't believe in God, being humble is a wise character trait during a life on this planet earth. If and when you achieve greatness, give God the glory.

2) Pray more: Begin your day basked in prayer and seek divine guidance can create a new inner desire to serve and boost your creativity. Realize where your help comes from, where your source of strength and creativity come from, and act accordingly. Begin realizing the greatness of God.

3) Begin reading scripture: I would recommend the Bible, as it is the source of tremendous knowledge, wisdom, and spiritual insight. Ask God to speak to you through it. Try this every day for 60 days and see what happens. You may be surprised!

4) Consider attending a church: Besides great spiritual knowledge and blessings that you receive from a church, you also benefit from a wonderful group of people who desire to befriend you, fellowship with you, and join you in a journey towards spiritual wellness. A church family can really be a source for inspiration for you.

If you are offended by the information above because it goes against your current faith, I apologize. I know we each find our own way to spirituality. This has been the road that God has taken me. I hope that it becomes yours as well, as it is filled with truth, love, and hope.

If you doubt the statements you have just read, or maybe you find some truth in them, but are uncertain where to go from here, I encourage you to begin investigating this subject deeper. The first and foremost authority is the Bible. Start there.

IMPORTANT NOTE! Please do not think that if you follow this spiritual path that you have to suddenly change your music style. **It doesn't mean you have to start a Christian rock band or start creating New Age Music.** If you do, that's great, but God created music in all forms. There are many great famous bands that are not Christian or new-age bands but are still spiritual in nature. There are many artists that you love and listen to on the radio every day that are very spiritual and godly people. They perform and sing in every genre; country, reggae, world music, rock, rap, etc. Bands like U2 spread a very powerful message to the masses. Just follow your heart where it leads you. God created music and he enjoys every rhythm and style that you offer back to him!

THE SPIRITUAL JOURNEY CONTINUES

Our spiritual journey never ends. Throughout our lives, we endeavor to become closer to God. As our heart changes and love is placed over old hurts, our relationship with God enhances. Don't miss out on the most beautiful aspect of being alive – finding and loving God.

Now, it's time to focus on restoring wellness when you've become injured. Let's move on to the next chapter.

Chapter Ten

RESTORING WELLNESS WHEN INJURED

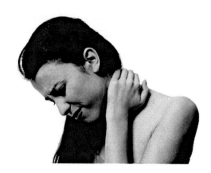

CONGRATULATIONS, YOU'VE NOW GAINED the tools to improve your mind, body & spirit. Although we are almost to the end of the book, I want to talk a bit about existing injuries in musicians and how to regain wellness and overcome pain and disability. Some of this information may seem repetitive from earlier chapters, but it is VERY important that we cover this subject in a little more depth. I would not be doing you justice if we did not search a little deeper. Here we go:

HOW BAD IS THE INJURY?

I've received hundreds of emails from musicians from all around the world, complaining about everything from fingertip pain to full-blown cervical spine disk injury with muscle weakening and severe pain. If you are experiencing a symptom of any magnitude, first ask yourself the question, "What is this symptom trying to tell me, and how can I learn from it?" Begin evaluating yourself for poor posture, technique problems, your diet, and your level of emotional stress. All these factors are typically causes for injuries developing in the musician.

I have found a common trait among musicians who have suffered repetitive strain injuries. It is the "I thought the pain would go away" concept. Many musicians are attempting to play their instrument, even though their arms, elbows, shoulders, neck, hips, or legs are experiencing pain or discomfort. You have to realize that pain is your body is a warning signal. It is like the engine light in your car going on. If your engine light goes on, hopefully, you don't ignore it, saying, "I hope that light goes off by itself. It can't be that important." That would be ludicrous, wouldn't it? You could wind up with a dead car alongside a long stretch of highway, wishing you had listened to the warning and taken care of it days or months ago. Yet this is what people do to their bodies all the time! They work through the pain signals, ignoring them, and expecting them to stop. When the symptoms don't stop, people become frantic wondering where to find a doctor to "fix" them.

Are you letting this happen to your body? Are you letting the signs and symptoms of a major malfunction in your body escalate to the point of total destruction? I'm sorry to say, that unfortunately, I see many musicians only once they've reached this point. They come in my chiropractic office in desperation, stating they can't play anymore because of the pain, and are afraid that their career is ruined. Don't let this happen to you!

To understand the injury, let's start by understanding why the body malfunctions. But first, you must understand some basic facts about how the body works.

1) Your nervous system (the brain, spinal cord, and all the nerves that branch off the spinal cord) controls EVERYTHING in your body. This includes muscles, organs, glands, tissues, cells, immunity, hormones, reproductive system, etc. Let's put it another way - there's nothing that occurs in your body without the brain controlling it.

2) The nerve system is the "life force" of the body. It literally supplies life to the muscles, tissues, glands, and organs. Without this life-supplying nerve input, your tissues disease and eventually die. Ever see what a spinal cord injury does to a person? That's a pure example of a deadened nerve system.

3) Insults to your body, in the form of physical stress, chemical stress, or emotional stress can "blow fuses" at the neurological fuse box - the spine. The medical terminology for these blown fuses is called a spinal subluxation. The spinal subluxation results from physical, chemical and emotional stress and creates irritation and distortion of the nervous system signals. A subluxation is a misalignment of a spinal bone(s) that exerts stress upon your nervous system. This leads to a distortion of nerve flow and abnormal signals reaching the tissues, organs, and glands.

4) Stress of all types will affect your entire body function. These continued stressors will eventually lead to symptoms due to difficulty or inability of the body adapting to the stress levels. This

leads to repeated stress on the neuro-spinal system eventually leading to disease, disability, and a shortened lifespan. Let's break down these types of stresses and how they relate to musicians in the following three stress producers:

- **Physical stresses**: (things that physically stress your body) Bad posture while playing your instrument, prolonged playing times without breaks, playing in one position (sitting for example) for a long time, previous car or motorcycle accidents, birth injuries (as a baby), previous sports injuries, quickly ramping up practicing times due to an upcoming gig or recital, being out of shape and overweight, sitting at computers for a long time, playing computer games hour after hour.
- **Chemical Stressors**: (things knowingly, or unknowingly put into your body), drugs and alcohol, prescription drugs, fast food, vaccine reactions, toxic chemicals in your environment (like chemicals you're exposed to by work or at home), a bad water supply, sugar substitutes, etc.
- **Emotional stressors**: (stuff you're thinking about) getting that recording contract, composing and finishing songs by a deadline, record company execs being a pain is the ***, family stresses, relationship stress, job stress other than your music career, death of loved ones, relocating, being on tour without family or loved ones nearby, and finally your negative thinking AKA "stinkin' thinkin'". I bet you never thought that all these things mentioned have a direct impact on your body!

Where are your weaknesses? What is "stressing" your body out? List them here so you can begin to improve yourself:

PHYSICAL STRESS

_____

_____

_____

_____

CHEMICAL STRESS

_____

_____

_____

_____

EMOTIONAL STRESS

_____

_____

_____

_____

So let's summarize in a real, practical situation that every musician can understand. You feel that you're in pretty good health, except for the fast food (chemical stress) that seems to be part of your lifestyle lately. You know that you're not eating right, but hey, there's this recording deal that you have to provide music for. You're spending eight to ten hours a day composing music, (physical and emotional stress) sitting at your guitar and piano. That certainly doesn't give you time to fix good meals. What's worse is that your girlfriend (or boyfriend) is hounding you because you don't spend enough time with them (which creates emotional stress). Your dad recently had a heart attack, and you're torn because you can't spend enough time with him right now, which produces more emotional stress. You're finding that one or two beers aren't sufficient anymore to handle your stress level. Drinking a six-pack is becoming part of your practice sessions. (Chemical stress) To top things off, your back is beginning to hurt after playing guitar for more than a few hours, so you begin taking some ibuprofen every day to make it through the sessions, which is adding more chemical stress.

What you're eating, talking, saying, doing, and hearing is impacting your current level of health. AN INJURY DEVELOPS WHEN THESE CON-TINUED STRESS FACTORS BEGIN TO BREAK DOWN YOUR NERVOUS AND SPINAL SYSTEM AND CAUSE YOUR MUSCLES, ORGANS, AND GLANDS TO ENTER A DISEASED STATE.

So, let's consider your injury at this point in time. Look back at this list of stressors and see which ones you've experienced lately; and it doesn't have to be within the past month or two. This list can go back to birth! Complicated you say? You're right. When a musician walks in my office with a repetitive injury, we have to investigate that entire person's life to find out what stressors led him/her to this current symptom. In many cases, even though the pain is in the arm, the actual nerve stress that is leading to the symptom can stem anywhere from the brain stem, neck, upper back, all the way to the lower back and even the feet. You have to investigate the whole body.

For deep rooted neurological insults that have resulted from stress very early in life, for example from a troubled childhood, divorce of your parents, serious injuries as a child or adolescent, or chemical traumas such as vaccine damage, there are specialized chiropractic methods to help the body release even the deepest internal stress. In my practice, I use methods to help rid the brain and nervous system of disease-causing distortions and strain that have developed from physical, chemical, emotional, and even spiritual stress from the point of conception to current time.

So now that you understand better how the body functions and how it breaks down, you are probably wondering how can you begin repairing the damage? First, work at relieving stressors in your life. (That's not easy.) Second, if you think your life stressors have taken their toll on your body, then visit a chiropractor to determine if your nervous system malfunctioning. Third, if you are having active repetitive strain injury symptoms don't wait — run to a chiropractic office for a complete evaluation and treatment. For a list of chiropractors that have experience working with musicians, go to my web site:

www.musicianshealth.com/CPAN.htm.

THE DANGERS OF ALLOPATHIC MEDICINE

Would you entrust your health care to a system that kills nearly one million people per year, just in the United States alone? If I were to tell you that a certain type of drug has been shown to kill a million people per year, I'm sure you would stay far, far, away from that drug. But in the United States people flock to medical doctors for all sorts of health conditions and even seeking wellness when it is being shown that allopathic medicine is the NUMBER 1 KILLER in the U.S.! A decision to visit an MD for your health care can be life-threatening as you begin to truly understand the statistics shown on the chart below.

The information and charts that follow are from the article *Modern Health Care System is the Leading Cause of Death* (2004 publication) by By Gary Null

PhD, Carolyn Dean MD ND, Martin Feldman MD, Debora Rasio MD, Dorothy Smith PhD and from the website: www.mercola.com.

ANNUAL PHYSICAL AND ECONOMIC COST OF MEDICAL INTERVENTION

CONDITION	DEATHS	COST	AUTHOR
Adverse Drug Reactions	106,000	$12 billion	Lazarou[1] Suh[49]
CONDITION	DEATHS	COST	AUTHOR
Medical error	98,000	$2 billion	IOM[6]
Bedsores	115,000	$55 billion	Xakellis[7] Barczak[8]
Infection	88,000	$5 billion	Weinstein[9] MMWR[10]
Malnutrition	108,800	--------	Nurses Coalition[11]
Outpatients	199,000	$77 billion	Starfield[12] Weingart[112]
Unnecessary Procedures	37,136	$122 billion	HCUP[3,13]
Surgery-Related	32,000	$9 billion	AHRQ[85]
TOTAL	**783,936**	**$282 billion**	

It is important to understand that medicine is excellent at crisis care and critical emergency situations. Allopathic medicine *is* helpful in certain situations. For example, if you break an arm or leg or suffer from destroyed knee cartilage, a good orthopedist is indispensable. If you suffer a heart attack, a hospital ER doc can save your life. If you need plastic surgery because of a serious burn, a plastic surgeon can do wonders.

BUT, many people rely on today's "modern" medicine to promote health in their lives. Well, guess what, you cannot find health in a pill bottle or through a surgical procedure! Health comes from within, as we spoke before. Anytime you begin chasing pills, getting surgeries, drinking potions, or applying salves and ointments to enhance your health, you are destined to go down the path of sickness, disease, and destruction.

Fortunately, many of the new enlightened MDs are beginning to embrace natural health care, such as chiropractic, acupuncture, massage therapy, and homeopathy, because they understand that medicine has its limitations and its dangers.

As a musician, you must be knowledgeable about the inherent risk you take by going to a medical doctor for problems such as carpal tunnel syndrome, cubital tunnel syndrome, TMJ dysfunction, thoracic outlet syndrome, and even tendonitis! The philosophical constructs of medicine indicate that all symptoms are bad, and drugs should be used to stop or mask them. This is far from the truth, because you should listen to your symptoms and allow them to tell you where the true underlying cause of those symptoms is stemming from. Vitalistic healing arts like chiropractic and acupuncture seek to address the cause of dysfunction, rather than the symptoms. This is why these disciplines are much safer, involve no medications, and seek to clear the body of inner distress and disease by restoring its natural homeostasis.

Also realize that if you visit a surgeon about a disease process in your body, you are very likely to get surgery as a recommendation. (If you're a hammer, everything looks like a nail.) That's the "state-of-the-art" in medicine. If you go to a surgeon with tingling in the first three fingers of the hand, guess what! You are now a candidate for carpal tunnel surgery! Statistics even show us that there are certain parts of the United States that have higher amounts of spinal surgeries, independent of the entering complaints. So the current level of health care (or should we call it sickness care?) you receive depends upon your zip code! I've seen so many people go down this route with poor long-term benefit because the CAUSE was never addressed.

What if that tingling and numbness is being caused by spinal subluxations (misalignments) and irritation of the sensitive nerves that exit the spine in your neck? What if it is caused by a nutritional deficiency? It is going to be missed by the MD who will almost never evaluate the spine for carpal tunnel syndrome, and knows very little about nutrition. For this reason, everyone who has an evaluation by an MD or physical therapist should balance it out with a chiropractic evaluation as well.

In a perfect world, the vitalistic health disciplines and allopathic medicine should work together harmoniously. Yet this is still far off because of age-old philosophical wars that exist between the disciplines. There are still medically-based groups that try to squash anything vitalistic. For example, there are even medically supported websites that question anything that is conservative and vitalistic. You would think that in this day of enlightened minds and the wealth of information on the Internet showing the promise of natural healing, that these ridiculous propaganda machines would no longer exist. But they are still around and do quite a disservice to the public, continuing the "turf wars" that really are unnecessary in our current health market. The consumer has the right to choose who or where he/she will go for health care.

WHAT ABOUT OTHER ALTERNATIVE HEALING TECHNIQUES?

There are numerous options for someone seeking alternative (non-allopathic medicine) health care for their injuries. I continue to recommend chiropractic as your portal of entry into the health care system. But in addition to chiropractic, there are other options as well. I am not an expert in these areas and can only offer them to you as options. For example, acupuncture and acupressure are alternative methods often used by musicians to relieve pain, enhance microcirculation and balance the body's energy pathways. Another path some musicians take is bodywork techniques like Feldenkrais and Alexander Technique. These are both methods of enhancing posture and releasing strain upon the musculoskeletal system. For more information about alternative healing methods, consider my book *Repetitive Strain Injuries: Alternative Treatments and Prevention*. A link can be found for purchase of this book on my web site, musicianshealth.com or at various other websites such as Amazon.com.

Chapter Eleven

CONTINUING YOUR NEW HEALTH PARADIGM INTO THE FUTURE

THIS BOOK HAS GIVEN YOU TREMENDOUS insight into caring for your body. We covered physical, chemical, mental, and spiritual health and how it pertains to musicianship and bodily function. Implementing all the concepts in this book can seem a bit daunting at first. Before closing, I want to recommend an implementation program for you to get you started so you can begin the process of health enhancement and total wellness.

The first thing you should do is to sit down and fill out the table below. 0 would be the absolute terrible end of the spectrum, 5 would be average and 10 would be the excellent end. Check off the box that pertains to your current health level in each category.

	0	1	2	3	4	5	6	7	8	9	10
Body weight											
Sleep habits											
Posture											
Nutritional intake											
Water intake											
Avoiding sugar											
Exercise regularly											
Overall health											
Aerobic health											

Muscular health												
Self-esteem												
Goal setting												
Daily affirmations												
Financial stability												
Tithing and giving regularly												
Job stability												
Family stability												
Emotional stability												
Spirituality												
Church attendance												
Read the bible regularly												
Give thanks regularly												
Pray daily												

Anything you rate 7 and above would be considered a strong point for you. You don't need to work on those. But if you rate any of these areas 6 and below, then those are the wellness areas you need to focus on.

Start with the lowest scores first. For example, if you find that exercise is your weakest area, then set a goal to begin exercising and also set out an action plan with a date that you will begin. This might be joining the local health club tomorrow and begin a workout routine. If you have many physical problems that bring your "overall health" quotient down, then consider seeking some healers in chiropractic or acupuncture to begin enhancing your wellness. If you haven't stepped foot in a church for twenty years, find an exciting church in your neighborhood that is full of great programs and interesting preaching and try it out again.

Increase your spirituality and your mind and body will become enhanced along with it. The important thing is to take action now! Don't put this off until next week or next month. Start today! Your Time Is Now!

Even if you just take one or two action steps after reading this book, then you have accomplished a great deal in your life. You are heading toward a more wellness-oriented lifestyle that will pay great dividends in years to come. As your wellness quotient increases, you will begin to tackle other weaknesses on the list and take total charge of your life and health.

Congratulations on making those first steps toward a wellness lifestyle. You will not regret the decisions you make today. Keep this book with you in your gig bag (like I mentioned at the beginning of the book), adopt these attitudes as your lifestyle and watch your health, wealth and success soar!

Well, I hope you've enjoyed this book. Feel free to contact me with any questions you may have about optimizing health and wellness. My email can be found on the final page of this book. Keep in touch, let me know about your progress and I'll let you know when the next book is being released.

God bless,
TIMOTHY JAMESON

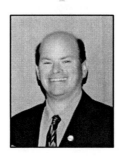

DR. TIMOTHY JAMESON graduated from Los Angeles College of Chiropractic in 1988 and has been in chiropractic practice ever since. He and his wife, Dr. Laurie Gossett, own Bayshore Chiropractic Family Wellness Center in Castro Valley, California, USA. (www.jamesonchiro.com) He specializes in working with the musician population and is the developer of an award-winning website addressing musician's health concerns, www.musicianshealth.com. The website won the Keyboard Magazine top 25 musician-related websites of the year in 2003. Dr. Jameson also founded the Chiropractic Performing Arts Network, a group of over 300 chiropractors who have an avid interest in enabling performing artists to reach their health care goals.

Dr. Jameson is heavily involved in the Christian music scene, providing on-site care for Christian performing artists as they pass through the San Francisco Bay Area. For many years he has provided backstage chiropractic care to musicians and stage crew at the three-day Spirit West Coast Christian music festival held yearly in Monterey, California.

Dr. Jameson's practice is family oriented and children-friendly. His practice philosophy is based on optimizing health and wellness for the entire family through chiropractic care, nutritional supplementation, exercise programs, reshaping mental attitudes, and encouraging people to seek higher levels of spirituality.

Besides chiropractic, Dr. Jameson enjoys his position as Worship Pastor at Christ's Community Church in Hayward, CA. He leads the team in vocals, and plays a D'Armond and Stratocastor electric guitar, and Martin and Yamaha acoustic guitars, and has a Yamaha S80 Synth keyboard. (Visit www.ccchayward.com to watch him lead worship through music.) He also enjoys gardening, making stained glass windows and Tiffany style lampshades, and digital photography.

He is married to wife Laurie, and is father to daughter Jillian and son Paul.

CONTACT INFORMATION:
Timothy Jameson, D.C.
3319 Castro Valley Blvd.
Castro Valley, CA 94546
510-582-5454

www.jamesonchiro.com
www.musicianshealth.com
email: chiro4u@aol.com

Seeking a consultation/treatment with Dr. Jameson? Contact Dr. Jameson by email or phone and discuss the possibility of visiting his office for evaluation and treatment of your injuries. He can also travel to your performance venue, studio, or internationally.

Would you like Dr. Jameson to speak to your group or organization? Dr. Jameson is available to travel to your organization to provide a wellness-based presentation, to optimize performance, musicality, and life experience.

Lightning Source UK Ltd.
Milton Keynes UK
UKOW031840141112

202228UK00017B/150/P